Take Heart!

A PROVEN STEP-BY-STEP PROGRAM
TO IMPROVE YOUR HEART'S HEALTH

Dr. Terence Kavanagh

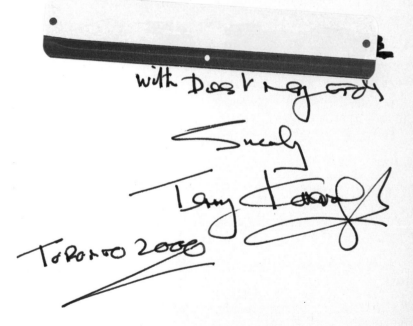

with Dear *illegible*

Sincerely

Terry Kavanagh

Toronto 2000

KEY PORTER BOOKS

Canadian Cataloguing in Publication Data

Kavanagh, Terence
  Take heart: a proven step-by-step program to improve your heart's health

Rev. ed.
ISBN 1-55013-970-3

1. Coronary heart disease —Prevention. 2. Heart —Diseases — Patients —Rehabilitation.
I. Title.

RC685.C6K38 1998   616.1'2305   C97-932718-0

The publisher gratefully acknowledges the support of the Canada Council for the Arts and the Ontario Arts Council for its publishing program.

THE CANADA COUNCIL | LE CONSEIL DES ARTS
FOR THE ARTS | DU CANADA
SINCE 1957 | DEPUIS 1957

Key Porter Books
70 The Esplanade
Toronto, Ontario
Canada M5E 1R2

www.keyporter.com

Illustrations and diagrams: Pages Design
Electronic formatting: Jean Lightfoot Peters

Distributed in the United States by Firefly Books

Printed and bound in Canada

98 99 00 01 02 6 5 4 3 2 1

Contents

Preface

Why a second edition of *Take Heart*!? One good reason is that the first edition was very well received by the lay public and health professionals alike; the other is that, since this book first appeared, we have learned a good deal more about coronary heart disease. For instance, any lingering doubt as to the wisdom of lowering high cholesterol levels has now been completely dispelled, due in large part to the effectiveness of the new cholesterol-lowering "statin" drugs. New risk factors have appeared on the scene, with strange-sounding names like homocysteine, chlamydia, and fibrinogen. There has been a greater recognition of the value of antioxidants in both the prevention and treatment of coronary heart disease, with our old friend vitamin E looking as if it might finally be coming into its own—possibly to be joined by a newcomer, coenzyme Q10. Abdominal obesity has now been identified as a trigger for a chain of coronary risk factors that include high blood pressure, elevated triglycerides, and Type II diabetes. The four, when seen together, are referred to as "The Deadly Quartet."

All of these developments are discussed in this new edition. I have also devoted more space to the topic of women and heart disease, and for good reason. More women die in the acute stages of a heart attack than men. Although a woman's long-term outlook after coronary artery bypass graft surgery is the same as a man's, the rate of immediate postoperative mortality is higher. The immediate results of angioplasty are not as good in women as in men. Some of the diagnostic tests used to detect coronary heart disease in men are less sensitive when used with women. As for the risk factors for coronary heart disease, most are the same as in men, although some, such as smoking and diabetes, are more dangerous. Unfortunately, we have failed to convince women of the dangers of heart disease and of the need to take action. More women are smoking today than ever. While men seem to be paying increased attention to their diet and their cholesterol level, women have yet to follow suit. Obviously we need to aim our heart-health-education programs more directly at women.

Not a month passes that we don't hear of a new study concluding that regular physical exercise is good for our heart. This was one of the main messages in the first edition, and it remains so in the second. For the patient with heart disease who does not have ready access to a formal cardiac rehabilitation program, this book provides a guide to a step-by-step safe and effective home training system, particularly if used in conjunction with advice from the family physician or cardiologist. Needless to say, healthy individuals who want to start exercising after years of sedentary living will also continue to find the home program and the section on self-fitness testing of considerable value.

As we approach the third millennium, it becomes apparent that coronary heart disease, a twentieth-century scourge, is destined to persist into the twenty-first century. Although we have seen a slow decline in the incidence of fatal heart attacks in North America and parts of Europe, in Eastern Europe and Asia, where junk food and a sedentary lifestyle are becoming the norm, the disease is escalating rapidly. It seems that if you live like a Westerner, you'll die like a Westerner. We can only hope the emerging industrialized nations will learn from our experience.

In the previous edition I gave a list of references at the end of the book. Apart from the fact that this is quite a chore, I've found that it was rarely used by readers. As an alternative, then, I have included the names of pertinent authors, articles, and journals in the text wherever I have felt them to be of particular importance.

As always, I am grateful to patients, colleagues, and staff alike who have made suggestions and advised me on the contents of this second edition. If you find it gives you a better understanding of heart disease and helps you achieve a healthier lifestyle, then you have them to thank.

1. A Modern Plague

Coronary heart disease has been called the twentieth-century plague and the World Health Organization has recognized it as our number-one killer. But despite this recent attention, the disease is not new. Examination of Egyptian mummies shows that it existed during the time of the Pharaohs, 3,000 years ago. Greek and Roman literature contains many references to what sound suspiciously like fatal heart attacks, that is, sudden death after the onset of severe chest pain. During the sixteenth and seventeenth centuries, when the Church lifted the ban against autopsies and they became the recognized method of determining the cause of death, more and more deaths were attributed to what we recognize today as coronary heart disease (CHD).

William Heberden, the eighteenth-century English physician, was the first to describe a symptom we now know to be an early manifestation of heart disease. Some of his patients, he said, "are seized while they are walking (more especially if it be uphill, and soon after eating) with a painful and most disagreeable sensation in the chest, which seems as if it would extinguish life if it were to increase or to continue; but the moment they stand still, all this uneasiness vanishes." He called this symptom angina pectoris (Latin for pain in the chest), and both the name and the description of the symptom have been used by doctors ever since. Although Heberden was unable to explain the precise cause of the symptom, he realized that it was associated with some form of heart disorder. Throughout his long life—and he lived until the age of 91—he faithfully recorded in detail each case he encountered. The fact that he accumulated only 100 such cases indicates that the condition was still relatively rare in the eighteenth century. Over the next hundred years, the theory slowly emerged that angina pectoris was caused by a disease process that *narrowed* the coronary arteries, the blood vessels that nourish the heart.

It was not until the early twentieth century that a Chicago physician, Dr. James Herrick, suggested that a heart attack was a later manifestation of the same process that caused angina pectoris, and that the heart attack was due to a *blockage* of a coronary artery. Herrick later commented on the fact that the scientific paper in which he first described this concept, published in 1912, aroused little interest among his fellow physicians at the time. Apparently in those days heart attacks were of less concern to doctors than they are today.

Currently, on a daily basis, heart attacks are responsible for some 1,500 deaths in the United States, 450 in the United Kingdom, and 120 in Canada. Approximately half these deaths occur in a matter of hours after the onset of chest pain, and often before the patient reaches hospital. In the United States, in addition to the one million people who suffer nonfatal heart attacks annually, 300,000 undergo coronary artery bypass graft surgery, 360,000 coronary angioplasty, and seven million suffer from angina pectoris. Initially a scourge of the Western industrialized countries, coronary heart disease is now also devastating the developing nations.

How did all this come about? It was once thought that the epidemic was more apparent than real, that doctors were simply diagnosing the cause of death with greater accuracy than their predecessors. Further investigation and observations on an international scale dispelled this theory and confirmed that heart attack mortality was on the increase. What had changed? Was it the population, the disease, or the environment? There is no evidence that human biology has changed, only a slight possibility that the disease has altered, and a good deal of evidence that it is our increasingly affluent lifestyle that is at fault. We will explore all of this later. In the meantime, let us take a closer look at the villain of the piece, known medically as a myocardial infarction, more commonly referred to as a heart attack.

PROFILE OF A HEART ATTACK VICTIM

John S. was entitled to feel pleased with himself. A professional engineer, at 41 he possessed all the contemporary hallmarks of success: a happy marriage, two teenaged boys who were doing well at school, a comfortable house (almost paid for) in a desirable neighborhood, and the prospect of promotion to company vice president. Mind you, he hadn't had too much time of late to count his blessings; a year previously the company plant started moving to a new location, and as production manager, he had found himself involved in a hectic work schedule. Even Mary, his usually patient wife, began to express concern as six- and seven-day work weeks became routine. Still, the job had to be done, and as he said, "Goodness only knows what a mess things would get into if I wasn't there to keep tabs on everything." Besides, when the move was completed, he could ease off a bit, perhaps "play a little golf, or take a week's vacation and get in a little fishing."

Maybe he would cut back on his smoking, too; with all the stress, he was up to a pack and a half a day now. It wouldn't do any harm to lose a little weight also, but that was difficult when one's meals consisted of an endless succession of sandwiches interspersed with "two-martini luncheon meetings" and expense-account dinners.

Yes, he probably was a little out of shape—which no doubt accounted for the heartburn and indigestion pain he had begun to experience in recent months whenever he got uptight at work or tried to lift anything heavy. He thought perhaps he was developing a peptic ulcer, the almost prestigious occupational disease of successful executives.

In due course, John's plant completed its move. But the transition brought with it problems that, naturally, only John could solve. Admittedly, weekends at the office were no longer routine (although they did occur from time to time), but the 12- and 13-hour workday became commonplace. Always a hard driver, he was now in hot pursuit of the presidency, and he dedicated himself to the task with all the energy and determination that had characterized his performance as one of the best linemen of his university football team. Unfortunately, he wasn't in his early twenties any more and, while he still possessed the spirit and motivation of bygone years, his body was no longer fit enough to perform the tasks he asked of it. His "indigestion" pain was bothering him more frequently now, and not only after eating. From time to time, he experienced severe discomfort in his upper abdomen and chest when he ran up a flight of stairs, or walked quickly up an incline (not that he did too much walking nowadays). Usually, the pain would go away if he belched or rested for a minute or so.

He began to feel chronically tired. Never at any time, however, did he feel that he had a serious health problem. He always came through the annual company medical examination with flying colors; blood pressure, electrocardiogram, blood and urine checks always normal—which was, after all, only to be expected in a strong, burly ex–college football player.

Then one day, while sitting dozing in front of the television set, he got a fright; the stomach pain came on quite suddenly. Only on this occasion it was more severe and seemed to have moved up into his chest. For a moment or two, he had difficulty breathing, as the pain radiated first into his neck and jaw, and then down both arms to his hands. He found he was sweating profusely. He didn't know what to do. When he tried to lie down, the pain seemed to get worse; moving around didn't do any good, and neither did belching. Mary, noticing his agitation and pale, sweating features, learned for the first time of his recurrent bouts of "indigestion." She wanted to call a doctor, but John persuaded her to wait and see if his condition improved. Fortunately (or unfortunately, as it turned out), the pain subsided after about 30 minutes, although for the next day or two his chest felt very sore. In deference to Mary's wishes, he called his family physician the following week and told him that he had been getting "the occasional niggling stomach pain when I am overtired or tense." A combination of John's natural tendency to downplay any evidence of physical weakness, together with what may have been a too-easy acceptance of his tale by the physician, led to a diagnosis of "nerves." An electrocardiogram was not carried out.

During the following weeks, John continued his heavy work schedule, suffering only occasional and relatively mild "nerve" pains in his chest—until the week the plant workers went on strike. If the job was hectic before, it was frenetic now. Extra duties, extra hours, unpleasantness on the picket lines, all contributed to a desperate situation. There seemed to be no solution. As a matter of fact, there was, and in John's case, it was almost the final one.

At four o'clock in the morning, he was awakened by the

most severe pain in his chest he had ever experienced. It was as if a terrible weight was pressing on his chest bone, squeezing and squeezing until he felt he could no longer breathe. He thought he was going to die. He put up no argument when Mary called the ambulance. Within half an hour, an electrocardiogram was carried out in the emergency department and the young, serious-looking doctor quietly gave him the news; he had sustained a severe heart attack and was to be admitted to the intensive care unit immediately.

John spent two weeks in hospital, during which time he experienced a series of emotional reactions to his predicament. At first, he was stunned by the doctor's diagnosis. It was impossible for him to have had a heart attack; his heart wasn't weak, he had never had a day's illness in his life—there must be some mistake. This period of denial lasted about 48 hours. Some patients never pass beyond it, even after discharge from hospital, persisting in their belief that the doctors have made a mistake. In John's case, it was replaced by a sullen anger. What right had fate to treat him in this unfair fashion? Hadn't he worked hard to make his mark in life, to provide for his wife and family, to get on? What reward was this for living according to the rules? Then he became depressed. Was he going to be an invalid for the rest of his life?

Finally, John went home. He was still in a depressed mood. The first day back in familiar surroundings was almost too much for him. He felt so fatigued he had to go to bed after only a few hours. He had lost his old aggressive self-confidence and was fearful of responsibility. Even after his return to work, ostensibly fully recovered, Mary was at first surprised and then perturbed to find that he continued to lean on her, reluctant to take the initiative in financial or domestic matters requiring a decision.

This state of affairs continued until his doctor, sensing a deterioration in the family relationship, had a talk with him and asked him if he would like to attend an exercise rehabilitation class that had recently been instituted at the Toronto Centre. John agreed. Later, he commented that the rehabilitation program was "like a lifebelt to a drowning man. It's the best thing since sliced bread."

Of course, there is no such thing as a typical heart attack victim. Patients come in all shapes and sizes. John's story is a composite case history, drawn from the files of patients referred to the Toronto Centre for post-coronary rehabilitation. Interestingly, our analysis of these patients, published in the *Canadian Medical Journal*, revealed a surprising similarity in the patterns of life prior to their heart attacks. Comparison with a matched group of healthy individuals showed that the patients who had sustained a heart attack also experienced a greater than average degree of business, financial, or domestic stress in the year prior to their illness. In many cases, the stress factor was extreme.

In the weeks before the attack, a significant number of them had experienced vague pains in the chest, neck, jaw, or arms, but had ignored these symptoms, ascribing them to indigestion or nerves. Most described a feeling of incredible fatigue, one man actually falling asleep while dining with a business client, and another instinctively reacting to the news of his heart attack with the thought, "At least I'll be able to get a good sleep at the hospital." Being overweight, heavy smoking, and lack of regular physical activity were all too common.

Not infrequently the attack itself occurred within 24 hours of a severe emotional experience or unaccustomed physical stress—for example, following a violent argument with the boss, or after half an hour of trying to start a stalled outboard motor. In at least one case, the emotional and physical were combined when a patient undertook a long and exhausting journey to see a boyhood house full of bittersweet memories.

Another study carried out at the Centre, also published in the *Canadian Medical Journal*, showed that many of these patients go through a phase of denial after the infarction, then all too frequently become depressed, lacking in confidence, and fearful for the future. The men feel they have lost their masculinity, and they worry about their ability to perform the role of husband and father with the same success as previously. Women victims feel a similar sense of insecurity, whether they are housewives or career-oriented. Both men and women hide their depression, even from their spouses, and it requires careful questioning by the physician and the psychologist to uncover it.

By now you should be getting a picture of the manner in which coronary artery disease can strike its victim, often an apparently healthy, busy man in his forties. Women of similar age are less frequently affected, and we will see the reason for this later. But what exactly is coronary artery disease, and what causes it? In order to answer these questions, we must take a brief look at the anatomy and physiology of the heart and blood vessels, and then make a short excursion into the field of epidemiology (the study of epidemics).

THE HEART: STRUCTURE AND FUNCTION

Situated in the center of the chest cavity, between the lungs, the heart is about the size of your clenched fist. In shape, it bears some likeness to the Valentine symbol, but there the resemblance ends. In structure and function, it is about as tender, delicate, and romantic as a sledgehammer. Its thick muscular walls surround a cavity that is divided into right and left sides by a longitudinal muscular partition, called the septum. Each side of the heart is further subdivided by a horizontal partition, which separates it into an upper thin-walled chamber, called the atrium

(Latin; entrance chamber), which receives the blood, and a lower thick-walled pumping chamber, called a ventricle (Latin; small belly), which ejects the blood. The right side of the heart receives the used, oxygen-poor blood from the body and pumps it through the pulmonary arteries to the lungs, where it is re-oxygenated. From the lungs, the oxygen-rich blood returns to the left side of the heart through the pulmonary veins. From here it is pumped through a large artery, called the aorta, to be distributed throughout the entire body. One-way valves between the atria and the ventricles prevent backflow into the atria when the ventricles are pumping. Similar one-way valves protect the mouths of the aorta and pulmonary artery, opening when the ventricles are pumping and closing when they are in the relaxation phase (Figure 1).

Thus, the heart functions as a pump—but what a pump! Beating an average of 72 times per minute, day and night, it circulates the body's entire blood volume of five to six liters within a minute. In a 24-hour period, it pumps an amazing 2,192 gallons (8,300 liters), or over 792,510 gallons (3 million liters) a year!

The sequence of events carried out by the heart is referred to as the cardiac cycle. It is divided into a pumping phase, when it is delivering blood around the body (known as the phase of systole), and a relaxing phase, when it is receiving blood returning from the body and the lungs (known as the phase of diastole) (Figure 2). When the heart is beating at its usual resting rate of 72 beats per minute, the systolic phase lasts about three-tenths of a second, and the diastolic phase five-tenths of a second. When the heart is beating much more quickly, for example during exercise, then both systolic and diastolic phases may be shortened by as much as 50%.

The environment of the planet Earth is unique (as far as we can tell to date). Its atmosphere consists of a mixture of gases containing 21% oxygen. Our bodies are

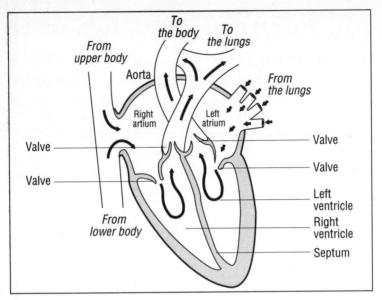

Figure 1: The Heart Pump
Four valves ensure that blood flows through the four chambers of the heart in one direction only.

designed to utilize that fact. If we are deprived of oxygen, the cells in our body begin to die, starting with the sensitive brain cells. Therefore, the mechanism by which we extract oxygen from the air and utilize it is of paramount importance. This mechanism, known as the "oxygen transport system," works in the following manner: A series of feedback systems throughout the body keeps the brain constantly informed of the level of oxygen in the bloodstream and the tissues. When the oxygen content falls below a critical level, the brain, acting through a relay of nerves, causes the diaphragm and the muscles between the ribs to contract. This increases the size of the chest cavity and creates a partial vacuum. Air is sucked into the expanding lungs and fills the tiny air sacs, or alveoli, of which there are literally millions in the lung tissue. Each alveolus is surrounded by a network of blood vessels called capillaries. When the air reaches the alveolus, it

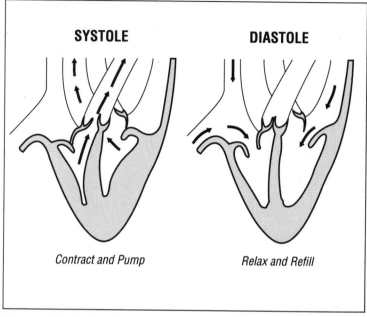

SYSTOLE   **DIASTOLE**

Contract and Pump   *Relax and Refill*

Figure 2: The Cardiac Cycle

releases its oxygen, which then passes through the thin alveolar and capillary walls into the bloodstream, where it combines with a protein in the red cell called hemoglobin (Figure 3). It is this combination, called oxyhemoglobin, that gives blood its bright red color.

The blood, now fully oxygenated, passes from the lungs through the pulmonary vein to the left atrium and then to the left ventricle. The left ventricle pumps the oxygenated blood out through the aorta into the arteries, which branch into smaller arterioles, and then finally into the even smaller capillaries that course throughout all the cells of the muscles and organs. Once in the capillaries, the blood gives up its life-sustaining oxygen and receives in return the carbon dioxide and other waste products produced by the working cells. This oxygen-poor blood, now referred to as venous blood, is carried back through the veins to the right side of the heart where, as we have seen,

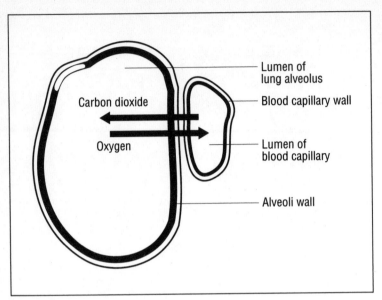

Figure 3: The Function of the Alveoli
Oxygen passes from air in the lung's alveoli to the blood in the capillary vessels through the two thin walls.

it is pumped to the lungs. Once there it gives off its carbon dioxide, picks up its supply of oxygen, and the cycle starts again (Figure 4).

The heart, therefore, is the driving force of the oxygen transport system, the pump that must keep working day and night in order for us to survive. All very well, you say, but nowhere in this description is mention made of the method by which the heart obtains its own supply of oxygen-enriched blood. Since the explanation is vital to our understanding of heart disease, we will need to describe this in some detail.

The Blood Supply of the Heart: the Coronary Circulation

The heart receives its oxygen-rich blood supply through the left and right coronary (crown-like) arteries (Figure 5). They emerge from the root of the aorta and are the first of the

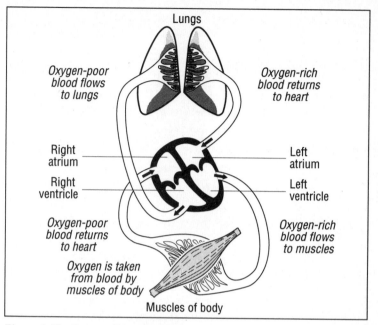

Figure 4: The Oxygen Transport System

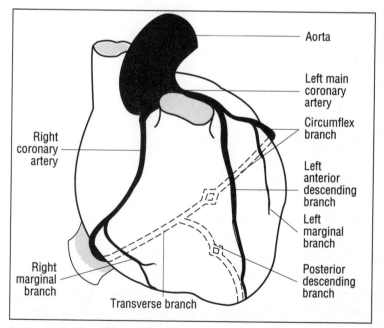

Figure 5: The Heart's Blood Supply – The Coronary Arteries

many branches that arise from that large arterial trunk as it passes down through the chest and abdomen to the pelvis.

The left coronary artery, referred to as the *left main*, arises from the back wall of the aortic root and then quickly divides into two branches, the *left anterior descending artery* and the *circumflex artery*. The left anterior descending branch runs down the front of the heart to the tip, or apex, then curves underneath and ascends the back wall for a short distance. The circumflex branch encircles the left side of the heart to the back wall, giving off a branch that descends along the left margin of the heart. Thus between them the left anterior descending and circumflex arteries supply blood to the front wall of the heart, its left margin, and its apex. Interference with the flow of blood through either of these branches, but particularly the left anterior descending, would obviously jeopardize a major area of heart muscle. A blockage occurring higher up, in the left main artery, would be even more critical, since it would cut off the blood flow through both the circumflex and anterior descending branches.

The *right coronary artery* arises from the front of the aortic root, curves around the right side of the heart to cross the back wall (as the *transverse branch*), where it meets the end of the circumflex artery. It also sends a *posterior descending branch*, which descends the back wall to meet the terminal portion of the left anterior descending artery. The right coronary artery supplies blood to the right side and back wall of the heart.

Because the left main artery is so short and branches so quickly, we often refer to three rather than two coronary arteries, that is, the right, the left anterior descending, and the circumflex. All these branches feed a network of blood vessels that penetrate the muscular walls of the heart, subdividing into arterioles and then capillaries, providing a rich blood supply to the highly specialized heart cells.

This, then, is the coronary blood supply, a system that

siphons off about one-twentieth of the blood that the heart pumps through the aorta every beat and redirects it back to nourish the heart itself. Considering its vital importance, the system should be problem free. Unfortunately, such is not the case. There are a number of flaws in the design, and they have a very definite bearing on the condition we now refer to as coronary heart disease.

The first problem has to do with the size of a coronary artery. Its inner diameter is not much larger than a drinking straw, and relatively minor encroachments on its inner wall can affect its ability to maintain a full flow of blood to the heart muscle. However, this would not matter so much if there were a rich, full, and plentiful network of interconnecting arteries linking the three main branches. Unfortunately, this is not the case. The connections, or collaterals, as they are called, are relatively sparse and tend to come into play only when considerable narrowing has already occurred in the main stem branches.

Thus, the heart's blood supply can be threatened by anything that reduces the flow of blood through its already small-bore coronary vessels. The culprit in CHD is a condition known as atherosclerosis, the medical term for a patchy plaque-like accumulation of fat that occurs in the walls of blood vessels. Atherosclerosis can affect any of the small- or medium-sized arteries of the body, whether in the brain (where it can cause a stroke), or in the legs (where it can lead to gangrene), or in the coronary arteries (where it can cause a heart attack). We will consider the nature and causes of coronary atherosclerosis later. For now, let us examine its consequences: angina pectoris, acute myocardial infarction, and sudden cardiac death.

THE THREE COMPLICATIONS OF CORONARY ATHEROSCLEROSIS

Angina Pectoris

As the coronary artery becomes narrowed by the protrusion of atherosclerotic plaques into its inner channel, or lumen, its ability to maintain a healthy supply of blood to the heart muscle gradually becomes impaired. For this reason, coronary heart disease is also referred to as ischemic heart disease, ischemia meaning "suppressing blood flow." In the early stages of coronary artery narrowing, or stenosis, there are no symptoms. This "silent" period is character-istic of the disease and may last for 20 to 30 years, depend-ing on the aggressiveness of the atherosclerotic process. We know from examination of young American soldiers killed in Korea and Vietnam, and young Israeli accident victims, that coronary disease can begin as early as age 20.

Ultimately, if the plaque grows so that it occupies more than 60% of the artery's inner diameter, blood flow through the coronary artery is so restricted that it cannot satisfy the demands of a fast-beating heart. Any number of things can cause the heart to beat faster: running, walk-ing up a hill, climbing stairs, sexual intercourse, even high emotional stress, such as an argument. When any working muscle is partially deprived of its blood supply, it develops a cramp-like pain. If you wrapped a tourni-quet around your upper arm so as to cut off the blood sup-ply, then clenched and unclenched your fist for a few minutes, you would soon develop severe pain in the muscles of your forearm. The pain would become increasingly worse until you were forced to stop making a fist. However, as soon as you released the tourniquet and allowed the blood to flow back into the forearm mus-cles, the pain would subside.

The heart muscle works the same way. Angina pectoris

is no more than cramp-like pain originating from the blood-starved, or ischemic, heart muscle. Classically, it is felt in the middle of the chest behind the chest bone. Patients may liken it to "a rope tightening around my chest" or "something heavy sitting on my chest." The pain may radiate up to the neck and down one or both arms. Typically it lasts for minutes, rather than seconds or hours, and gradually subsides when the sufferer ceases whatever activity brought it on. As you can see, this description doesn't add much to that given by Heberden over 200 years ago, a testament to his acute clinical observational powers.

A common situation in which both the emotional and physical factors occur together is the all-too-familiar struggle through one of our modern overcrowded airports while carrying a heavy suitcase. As soon as our anginal victim slows down or stands still, the work load on the heart is reduced; the narrowed coronary arteries can now supply enough blood requirements to the heart, and the pain goes away. Although repeated attacks of angina are to be avoided, and doctors prescribe medication to prevent them, they are not the same as a heart attack. Indeed, anginal symptoms may persist for many years without ever leading to the second manifestation of coronary artery disease: a heart attack. It is also important to understand that angina is due to a *temporary* shortage of blood to the heart muscle, which is corrected as the pain subsides, and does not cause any permanent damage to the heart.

Acute Myocardial Infarction (Heart Attack)

This term is used by pathologists and refers to the changes that occur in the heart muscle cells when they are permanently deprived of their blood supply. It represents a further stage in the progress of coronary atherosclerosis. At this stage, the narrowed coronary artery becomes completely blocked, and the portion of heart muscle it supplies loses its blood supply and dies (Figure 6). The block may

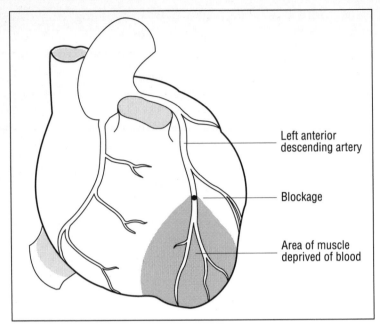

Figure 6: A Heart Attack

arise as the result of an atherosclerotic plaque gradually enlarging so that it eventually fills the lumen. In this case, the patient will have a lengthy history, maybe years, of increasing anginal pain at lower and lower levels of exertion before experiencing a heart attack. Not infrequently, however, there is no history of angina, just a sudden heart attack occurring in an apparently healthy individual. What is the mechanism here? We now know that the most dangerous phase in the development of an atherosclerotic plaque is its early stage. It is too small to restrict blood flow and cause angina, but it is very susceptible to rupture. If this happens, it discharges its contents of liquid fat into the bloodstream. The make-up of blood is 50% water, and since water and fat don't mix, a clot forms instantly. If the clot is large enough, it blocks the entire artery, cutting off blood flow, and resulting in a sudden heart attack.

Death of heart muscle tissue is responsible for the classical symptoms of a heart attack. The patient complains of severe and continuous chest pain that, unlike angina, does not go away, even when he or she stops all activity and rests. There are all the signs of shock: sweating, pallor, slow pulse rate, and falling blood pressure. Within a few hours, the electrocardiogram tracing becomes abnormal because the electrical signals from the heart muscle are being modified by the presence of dying tissue. There is also a rise in the blood level of various substances released by the breakdown of heart muscle tissue. These are known as enzymes; their diagnostic importance lies in the fact that they can often be detected by special laboratory tests prior to the appearance of changes in the electrocardiogram.

If the damage is severe, then the heart may stop beating ("cardiac arrest" or "ventricular fibrillation"), and the attack is fatal. If cardiac arrest occurs when the patient is already in hospital, then normal rhythmic beating may be restored by applying an external electrical current to the chest wall. This procedure is known as defibrillation. Obviously, there is a great advantage to having the patient in the intensive care unit; here the heart can be monitored continuously, and if cardiac arrest occurs, defibrillation can be carried out within seconds. Unfortunately, cardiac arrest is most likely in the first few hours of the attack, when decisions are still being made to call a doctor or arrange admission to hospital.

In recent years, a new form of treatment called thrombolytic therapy has been developed. In selected cases, and provided the patient is seen early enough after the onset of the heart attack, anticlotting substances are injected into the bloodstream to dissolve the clot in the blocked artery, restore normal blood flow, and reduce the extent of damage to the heart muscle. This will be discussed later.

Occasionally, when the area of damage is large, the pumping action of the heart may be compromised, and the patient is referred to as being in heart failure. Nowadays, with the advent of new and more powerful antifailure medications, the outlook for patients who develop heart failure is greatly improved.

Sudden Cardiac Death

This third and most devastating manifestation of coronary artery disease is one of the major problems facing medical science today. It is defined as death occurring shortly after the onset of heart attack symptoms in a patient who is apparently healthy and who, up to that point, never had any symptoms of heart disease. When I tell you that sudden cardiac death accounts for about 50% of all heart attack deaths, you will get some idea of the magnitude of the problem. Autopsy invariably shows advanced coronary artery disease, even though previous symptoms have been absent.

CHD IN WOMEN

The three clinical complications of CHD—angina pectoris, heart attack, and sudden cardiac death—occur in women as in men. Women tend to be protected from coronary heart disease during their childbearing years, but after menopause, natural or surgical, they catch up to the men very rapidly. So rapidly, in fact, that they are then more likely to die from a heart attack than they are from any other cause, including cancer. The sad thing is that while we have a lot to learn about the cause and prevention of cancer, we know quite a lot about the prevention of heart disease. If we were more successful in getting that knowledge across to women and persuading them to act on it, we would probably be able to cut their incidence of fatal heart attack by as much as 50%. In the United States, some 250,000 women die from coronary disease each year; the figure for Canada is 20,000. This problem deserves a section to itself, and will be dealt with in more detail in Chapter 3.

STROKE

Atherosclerosis is the commonest cause of a stroke, a condition in which part of the brain is damaged as a result of being permanently deprived of its blood supply. Depending upon the extent and location of the brain injury, there is loss of speech, memory defect, behavioral disorders, and full or partial paralysis of either side of the body. Fortunately, with specialized rehabilitation, the outlook for full or partial recovery can be good.

Strokes are of three types; cerebral hemorrhage, cerebral infarction, and cerebral embolus. *Cerebral hemorrhage* is due to rupture of an artery in the brain, with leakage of blood into the surrounding tissue. The cause of the break is weakness of the vessel wall, sometimes congenital, but usually as a result of atherosclerosis, combined with high blood pressure.

In a *cerebral infarction*, the artery is blocked by a blood clot on the rough surface of an atherosclerotic plaque. This type of stroke is also known as an "ischemic stroke."

The blockage may also originate in a clot located elsewhere in the body—the legs, lungs, or heart. A small piece of the clot breaks off and migrates through the blood vessels to lodge in the brain. The migrating clot is called an embolus, and this type of stroke is called an *embolic stroke*.

Strokes are the third leading cause of death in the advanced countries. They are more common in those over the age of 55 and are one and a half times more prevalent in men than women. For some reason, the incidence of strokes has not escalated as dramatically during this century as that of heart attacks.

2. What Causes Atherosclerosis?

The specialist writing for the nonspecialist reader is faced with the problem of presenting the subject as simply as possible without sacrificing fundamental accuracy. Obviously, too much attention to technical detail will make for tedious reading. On the other hand, oversimplification often leaves more questions unanswered than answered, or leads to confusion. The subject of heart disease and atherosclerosis is a case in point. In an attempt to educate the public, many health authorities have presented the disease in simplistic terms. Although I applaud their motivation, I cannot help but feel that this approach leads to problems of credibility down the line.

Almost everyone these days realizes that a heart attack is due to a blockage of a coronary artery. Many are even familiar with the term atherosclerosis. At this point, however, matters become oversimplified. Atherosclerosis is conceived as a blob of cholesterol sticking to the inner wall of the coronary artery. This blob is blamed on too much cholesterol in the blood, which, in turn, is blamed on eating foods high in cholesterol. Haven't we all been advised that too much cholesterol in our food or in our blood is dangerous? Mind you, many of us are not quite sure what cholesterol is, except that it is present in eggs and is presumably yellow in color. We also know from the labeling on food packages that any food that is "cholesterol-free" is safe to eat because it cannot give you heart disease.

If all of this is true, where does cigarette smoking enter the picture, or high blood pressure (doesn't that cause strokes)? What about diabetes, or stress, or family history, or lack of exercise? And then again, if we are merely dealing with fatty blobs that are "furring-up the pipes," why can't we just inject something like a medical form of Drano into the coronary artery to dissolve them? And what about those of us who have relatives or friends who consume prodigious amounts of fat, or smoke to excess, and yet live into their eighties or nineties? And finally, why do we continually read conflicting reports about the connection between heart disease and hydrogenated margarine, and even viral infections? Sound familiar? With all these questions unanswered by the initial simplistic concept of coronary artery disease, is it any wonder that many healthy young adults are still skeptical about what they are told and remain reluctant to stop smoking, reduce the amount of fat in their diet, exercise regularly, etc.?

On the other hand, if we start with the atherosclerotic lesion itself, then examine the various theories that have been proposed to explain its presence in the coronary arteries, we may get a better understanding. I will do my best to make the following as simple and as accurate as the subject demands.

Remember the famous real estate dictum that the three most important features in selling a house are location, location, location. So it is with atherosclerosis. The first key to understanding the condition is to have a clear idea of where it occurs. It's a popular misconception that an artery resembles a simple pipe. On the contrary, the walls of the coronary artery, like those of all arteries, are composed of three coats (Figure 7). The *inner coat*, or endothelium, consists of a single layer of smooth cells, called endothelial cells, over which the blood flows, and a surrounding sleeve of elastic tissue, which allows the endothelium to expand and then recoil so as to accommodate to the pulsations caused by the heart's pumping action. The *middle coat*, the thickest of the three, consists of smooth muscle fibers (so called because they are less complex in appearance than the coarser muscle fibers found elsewhere in the body), mixed with elastic fibers. This muscle layer can increase or reduce the flow of blood through the artery by constricting (vasoconstriction) or dilating (vasodilation) its diameter. Finally, there is a tough *outer coat*, which consists of a combination of elastic and connective tissue. This layer supports the nerves that control vasoconstriction and vasodilation, as well as the tiny blood vessels that supply nutrition to the inner two walls. The inner channel, through which the blood flows, is referred to as the *lumen*.

The mechanism by which the atherosclerotic lesion, or atheroma, involves these three walls is at the very heart (pardon the pun) of the debate over the cause of coronary heart disease. The term atheroma is a very old one. It is derived from two Greek words that, loosely translated, mean a tumor containing a porridge or gruel-like substance. In the past, it was used to refer to almost any tumor that contained a material of soft consistency. Only during the nineteenth century did it become associated specifically with the type of nodule or tumor that involves the walls of an artery. The most striking aspect of these nodules was that, when they were cut open, they were seen to contain a soft fatty material. Thus, the term atheroma seemed appropriate. When it was further recognized that a later stage in the growth of the atheroma involved the development of harder scarlike tissue, and even calcium, the term atherosclerosis (fatty hardening) was coined.

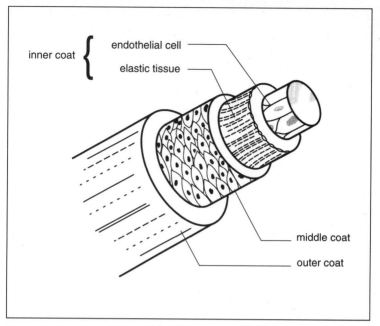

Figure 7: The Artery Wall with Its Three Coats

An atherosclerotic deposit large enough to reduce blood flow through the artery is seen by the naked eye as a raised, pearly-gray nodule that projects from beneath the endothelium into the lumen of the artery. Examining it in cross-section and under the microscope, we see that it also can extend through to the middle layer, and in very advanced cases, even into the outer layer of the artery. The pearly-gray cap consists of scarlike fibrous tissue. Beneath the cap is a disorganized collection of smooth muscle cells that have migrated from the middle layer into the inner layer, as well as a type of white blood cell known as a "scavenger" cell. The scavenger cells contain large amounts of fat. Fat is also seen in its free liquid form in the spaces between the scavenger and smooth muscle cells. Additional contents of the lesion include flakes of calcium, as well as the remnants of cells which have lost all recognizable shape (Figure 8). In addition to invading the

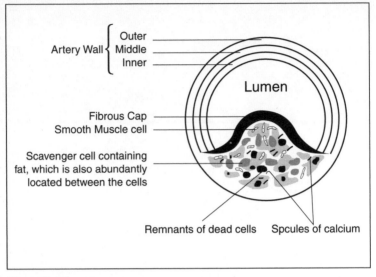

Figure 8: Atheroma

An atheroma with its contents. Note how it has invaded all three coats of the coronary artery wall and also projected into the artery's lumen, thereby obstructing blood flow.

walls of the coronary artery, the nodules can spread sideways, involving long segments of the vessel.

So much for the lesion itself. What about the mechanism responsible for its presence? It is now generally accepted that the first stage in the development of atherosclerosis is injury to the artery's smooth endothelial lining. Early animal experiments in which the endothelial cells were intentionally damaged with an instrument passed into the coronary artery resulted in a number of responses. The first response involved a type of blood cell called a platelet. Platelets are tiny round cells, about half the size of a red blood cell, that circulate in the blood in large quantities. If there is a cut in the blood vessel wall, they prevent bleeding by gathering in clumps, sticking to the vessel wall, and forming a clot that plugs the hole. However, platelets are incapable of distinguishing between a break in the smooth cellular endothelial lining and a cut which

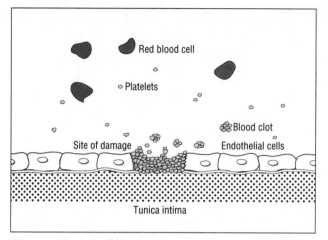

Figure 9: The Role of Platelets in the Formation of an Atheroma
Blood platelet cells stick to damaged endothelial lining of artery, clump together, and form a blood clot in an attempt to seal off break in the vessel wall.

extends through all three walls. As they clump around the injured endothelium, they not only cause a clot *inside* the artery, they release a substance that inflames the smooth muscle cells of the middle coat (Figure 9). As a result, the inflamed smooth muscle cells multiply, then overflow into the inner coat, where they combine with fat-laden cells to form an atheroma.

The Causes of Atherosclerosis
The next question is clearly: what causes injury to the endothelium? The three major risk factors that have been linked consistently to heart disease are cigarette smoking, high blood pressure (hypertension), and high blood cholesterol (hypercholesterolemia). How do these cause injury? Cigarette smoke contains many chemicals that can damage the endothelial cells. Chronic high blood pressure could also disrupt the endothelial layer by mechanical force alone, particularly at the areas where the arteries bend or branch—which is precisely where most atherosclerotic deposits are found. It is not so obvious how an

excess of cholesterol or fat in the blood damages the lining cells. On the other hand, substantial evidence has built up over the years suggesting that hypercholesterolemia does play a major causal role in coronary heart disease. Indeed, many proponents of the cholesterol theory maintain that it is the only cause. If the endothelial injury theory is correct, where does cholesterol fit in?

The answer has been sought in animal experiments. When blood cholesterol levels are high, the cholesterol particles are picked up by the scavenger white cells in the blood, and these cells then pass through the apparently intact endothelium where they accumulate as a "fatty streak." With continued transport of cholesterol-laden scavenger cells into the vessel wall the fatty streak grows in size, then ruptures through the overlying endothelial covering. The break in the endothelium then attracts platelets, which then initiate the inflammatory response that leads to an atheroma. Currently, this theory appears to fit the clinical facts. We will deal with this in more detail in Chapter 4.

SCIENTIFIC STUDIES

In order to understand the studies and trials on which our knowledge is based, an understanding of the terminology is necessary.

Retrospective studies identify patients suffering from a disease and, through medical interviews and examinations, attempt to discover which characteristics they have in common. For example, in the case of coronary disease, the common characteristic might be male gender or cigarette smoking; these are referred to as risk factors for coronary disease.

The predictive accuracy of risk factors established by retrospective studies can be tested by *prospective studies*.

These identify healthy individuals who possess the proposed risk factors, then follow them to see if they eventually develop coronary disease. Both types of studies make
no attempt to affect the outcome; they are purely observational in nature. Probably the best-known, and certainly
the most-often-quoted prospective study in the field of
coronary disease, is the U.S. Department of Health's
Framingham Study, which started in 1949 and is still
active (as one of its principal investigators, Dr. William
Kannel has said "It's a race to see who survives the
longest, the investigators or the investigated!").

In contrast, *clinical trials* test the effect on a disease of
some form of intervention—either drug, diet, or even regular exercise. In order to avoid biasing the results by inadvertently preselecting a group of subjects who might
respond favorably to the intervention, a process known as
randomization is used. Candidates for the trial are randomly allocated, usually by computer, to either a treatment or nontreatment (control) group. In the case of a
drug clinical trial, the control group is generally given a
placebo, an inert, harmless substance identical in appearance to the drug. This corrects for the placebo effect, a
well-known medical phenomenon in which some subjects
experience a benefit from any form of treatment merely
because they expect one. Since subjects do not know
whether they are taking the active drug or the placebo, the
trial is described as "blind."

When we come to evaluate the results of a clinical trial,
we need to compare the occurrence of a predetermined
measure, called the end-point, in the treated and the control groups; for instance, the occurrence of death from a
heart attack. However, we have to be sure that any difference in end-points between the two groups is not due to
chance. This is solved by subjecting the numbers to *statistical significance testing*. For a trial to show a statistically significant and conclusive result, the probability of any

difference in end-point between the treated and the control subjects happening purely by chance alone must be 5%
or less, expressed as p (probability) = 0.05. A probability
of more than 5% (p = 0.06 or greater) means a non-
significant or chance result. Obviously a probability of 1%,
or one in a hundred (p = 0.01), or of 0.1%, one in a thousand (p = 0.001) confers upon the difference in end-point
even greater statistical significance, and therefore makes
it even more conclusive.

Sometimes a trial may fall just short of achieving a statistically significant result, possibly because of method-
ological problems, e.g., not enough subjects were
recruited, or the time allowed for follow-up was too short.
In cases such as this, if the data from similar trials are
available, then we can resort to a statistical tool known as
meta-analysis. Here we pool all the results and analyze
them as if they came from a single trial. In this way we may
be able to detect from a series of "almost successful" trials an outcome which may be more conclusive. The use of
meta-analysis is rapidly increasing as we come to rely
more and more on clinical trials to prove, or disprove, the
value of various medical treatments.

By now you should have a better understanding of
coronary artery disease. We have reviewed its history, followed its disastrous path into the twentieth century, examined some theories as to its origins and causes, and
outlined the methods we utilize to detect and deal with it
in the community. The time has now come to talk about
who gets heart disease, why, and what can we do about it.

3. Risk Factors

The studies that have been carried out over the past 50 years have identified certain major characteristics and personal habits which increase the risk of developing atherosclerosis. These so-called "risk factors" can be subdivided into non-modifiable and modifiable (Figure 10).

Hypercholesterolemia and sedentary lifestyle will each be dealt with in separate chapters. This chapter will consider the two major non-modifiable risk factors—gender and heredity—then the remaining modifiable factors, as well as other possible factors which have been considered or are currently under investigation.

GENDER

Coronary artery disease is often referred to as a man's disease. This is more than a little unfair. We have seen in the previous chapter that it takes a heavy toll on women, particularly older women. In fact, the 3,000-year-old Egyptian mummy I mentioned earlier that was found to have a severe blockage of one of the coronary arteries was that of a 50-year-old woman. So why is coronary artery

MAJOR RISK FACTORS	
Non-Modifiable	**Modifiable**
Gender	High blood cholesterol
Heredity	(hypercholesterolemia)
	Sedentary lifestyle
	High blood pressure
	(hypertension)
	Diabetes
	Smoking
	Environmental stress
	and personality
	Obesity

OTHER POSSIBLE RISK FACTORS
Fibrinogen
Homocysteine
Bacterial and viral infections

Figure 10: Factors That Increase the Risk of Heart Disease

disease thought to be a man's problem?

The answer is to be found in the data obtained from the study of death rates from heart disease. If we examine the death rates from strokes in men and women over the period from 1900 to 1970, we will see that the ratio of male to female deaths does not change. However, from the 1920s on there was a steady increase in the number of males compared with females dying from heart attacks, the overall ratio increasing to as high as 3:1. What's more, most of the men dying were between the ages of 35 and 65. The current epidemic of heart disease thus commenced in the 1920s, and mostly attacks men in their middle years.

This evidence raises some questions. Why are men more susceptible, and why only since the 1920s? Does the female of the species have some gender-related factor that gives her an immunity from the epidemic?

Female Hormone

Pathologically, the lower incidence of coronary deaths in women is explained by the finding that, when matched for age, women have considerably less extensive coronary atherosclerosis than men. The probable explanation is that the female hormone estradiol, a form of estrogen pro-duced by the ovaries, protects women from the develop-ment of coronary atherosclerosis during the child-bearing years. After menopause, estradiol production falls and is replaced by the less active estrogen, estrone, which is pro-duced by non-ovarian tissue; the rate of atherosclerosis formation in women then increases.

In recent years, there has been an increasing tendency to prescribe estrogen therapy (ERT), or a combination of estrogen and progestin (HRT) for post-menopausal women in order to relieve symptoms such as hot flashes, to prevent osteoporosis and fractures, and to reduce the incidence of coronary heart disease. This practice is not as yet universal and physicians who do prescribe replace-ment hormones do so selectively, judging each patient individually and choosing for treatment those least likely to develop dangerous side-effects.

Nevertheless, if we want to explore the question of female hormone and immunity from heart disease, it seems only reasonable to look at the incidence of heart dis-ease in women receiving hormone replacement therapy. The majority of observational studies of these women show that post-menopausal estrogen users are at less risk for coronary disease. Dr. Stampfer and his colleagues from the Harvard Medical School studied 122,000 nurses in the Nurses' Health Study. The incidence of coronary events, fatal and nonfatal, in postmenopausal women taking estro-gen was less than half that occurring in non–estrogen users over the ten-year period of observation. Other similar stud-ies have confirmed these findings. On the other hand, there is compelling evidence that ERT can increase the risk of uterine cancer. This hardly matters if it is given to a woman who has had a hysterectomy; otherwise the risk can be reduced, if not eliminated entirely, by switching from ERT to an estrogen/progestin preparation, or HRT.

There have been conflicting reports on the incidence of breast cancer in women using HRT. The Nurses' Health Study reported a 30–40% increase in this disease, with the greatest risk in women aged 60 years and older and who had been using the hormone for more than five years. On the other hand, a study from the University of Washington involving 537 women with newly diagnosed breast cancer found no increased risk among women taking hormone therapy for eight years or longer. If anything, long-term use of HRT was associated with a *decreased* risk of breast cancer. So far, then, the evidence regarding HRT and breast cancer risk remains inconsistent. A definitive answer can be obtained only by prospective, randomized clinical trials which involve large numbers of both healthy women and those already suffering from coronary artery disease. Fortunately, two such trials are already underway, the Women's Health Initiative (WHI), which is a United States government-sponsored study, and the Heart and Estrogen/Progestin Replacement Study (HERS), a United States industry-sponsored trial. Results from the latter should be available by the end of the century; the WHI is designed to continue for some 12 to 15 years.

Assuming that the female hormone does have a protective effect, we still have to explain how it works. We know that estrogens change the levels of the different types of cholesterol found in the blood. As you will learn later, cholesterol can occur in two different forms, low-density lipoprotein cholesterol, LDL-C, and high-density lipoprotein cholesterol, HDL-C. A high level of LDL-C is associated with coronary disease. In contrast, a high level of HDL-C protects from coronary disease. The effect of estrogens is to increase blood levels of HDL-C and at the same time decrease LDL-C levels. As a result, women in their reproductive years have higher levels of HDL-C than men. This differential diminishes after the menopause. The question arises, therefore, whether hormones given after the onset of the menopause can prevent these adverse changes in cholesterol levels. This was answered by a large study, the Post-menopausal Estrogen/ Progestin Intervention Trial (PEPI) from the National Heart, Lung, and Blood Institute in the United States. It showed that although estrogen alone (ERT) gave HDL-C levels the largest boost, combined estrogen/progestin (progestin in both its synthetic and natural forms) also raised HDL-C and lowered LDL-C. Since estrogen/progestin was not associated with any precancerous changes in the uterus, this is obviously the preferred form of treatment. In addition, HRT decreased clotting tendencies in the blood, thus reducing the risk of a heart attack, and was shown not to be associated with any increase in blood pressure or gain in body weight.

The Pill

Another aspect of the female hormone puzzle concerns the birth control pill. During the 1980s, a number of reports linked heart disease with the use of the pill. Since the pill suppresses the function of the ovaries, using a combination of synthetic estrogen and its "antagonist," progestin, this result was not altogether unexpected. Once again there were confounding variables, such as a history of smoking, or the influence of aging. Smokers who were on the pill were reported to have as much as ten times the risk of a heart attack or stroke as nonsmokers, with the risk even higher in those over the age of 40. However, with time it became apparent that even more variables had to be taken into account. These included cholesterol levels prior to going on the pill, exercise habits, alcohol intake, the use of other medications, and so on.

Eventually, we have come to understand that it was the synthetic progestin in the pill that caused the increased incidence in heart attacks, but that this increase was relatively slight. Thereafter, pills were devised in which the amounts of progestin and estrogen were more evenly balanced. Finally, progestins were synthesized that do not harm the cardiovascular system. A report from the Royal College of General Practitioners in the United Kingdom shows that birth control pills currently in use increase coronary risk only in those users who are heavy smokers. However, the heavy smokers were found to have 20 times the risk of CHD as nonsmokers!

The Major Risk Factors and Gender
Even though younger women possess some gender-linked protective factor, we are still left with the unhappy statistic that coronary heart disease accounts for 250,000 deaths each year among American women. It is the third leading cause of death in women aged 35 to 39 years, the second in those aged 40 to 64 years, and first in women aged 65 and over. However, because of the greater male-to-female ratio of cardiac deaths in the age group 35 to 54, most of the research into the causes of coronary disease has involved men only. After all, if you want to learn as much as you can about a disease, it makes good sense to start by observing the group in which it is most prevalent. In short, you fish where there are the most fish. Or, as a famous bank robber replied when asked why he robbed banks, "Because that's where the money is."

But is it valid to assume that the conclusions gained from these studies on men also apply to women? In particular, do the same risk factors apply? With certain reservations, the answer would appear to be yes. What are these reservations?

Diabetes is a powerful risk factor in women. Women diabetics have a four- to sixfold risk of developing heart disease compared with nondiabetic women; men with diabetes have a twofold risk compared with nondiabetic men. In effect, diabetes completely erases the protective effect from coronary disease that women enjoy in their premenopausal years.

Younger women, often in their teenage years, are smoking in increasing numbers, possibly because they consider it "trendy" or because they fear gaining weight; yet cigarette smoking is a particularly dangerous risk factor for women under the age of 50 years. In this age group, those who smoke more than 15 cigarettes a day are four and a half times more likely, and those who smoke more than 30 cigarettes a day, ten times more likely to suffer a heart attack than nonsmokers. In fact, even women who are "light smokers" (one to four cigarettes daily) have more than twice the risk of coronary artery disease than nonsmokers. In short, the woman who smokes like a man will die like a man—or even more so! As in men, ex-smokers appear to be at little or no risk. Unfortunately, the evidence is that women find it harder to stop smoking than men. If, in fact, smoking is more addictive in women than in men, then we should be targeting women, and in particular younger women, in our antismoking campaigns. On the other hand, if the woman stops smoking, but the spouse doesn't, she is still at a 20–30% risk for a heart attack from inhaling second-hand smoke. And finally, as we have seen, smokers who are on the pill have as much as 20 times the risk as nonsmokers on the pill. This may have to do with the fact that cigarette smoking alters the estrogen metabolism in premenopausal women. The resulting lower estrogen levels cause premature menopause, which in itself increases the risk of coronary heart disease. All in all, because of the high prevalence of smoking among women, eliminating this habit would probably be the single most effective method of reducing their incidence of heart disease.

Hypertension is now recognized to be a strong risk factor for coronary heart disease in women, and yet 30% of
women over the age of 65, the age group most susceptible
to heart disease, are hypertensive. Studies in Australia,
Europe, and the United States have also demonstrated
that appropriate treatment results in a significant reduction in death from stroke and heart disease in patients up
to 84 years of age, with women benefiting to the same
degree as men.

We will examine the influence of blood cholesterol levels on coronary disease in more detail in Chapter 4. Suffice
it to say at this stage that in men there is a strong association between high total blood cholesterol levels and coronary heart disease. Does the same apply to women? The
answer seems to be yes, except that there is a greater need
to look at two other measurements, namely high density
lipoprotein cholesterol (HDL-C), the "good" cholesterol,
and triglycerides, the other form in which fat is carried in
the blood. Premenopausal women have more of their cholesterol in the HDL form than men, and therefore a total
cholesterol reading which would be considered a risk for
a man may not be for a woman, for the simple reason that
it is counterbalanced by the high HDL-C content. After
menopause, however, when estrogen production begins to
fail and HDL-C levels fall, then that same total cholesterol
reading becomes a risk factor. HDL-C readings are therefore essential in women if we are to interpret the importance of the total cholesterol measurement. High
triglycerides, often associated with obesity and diabetes,
when they are accompanied by low levels of HDL-C, may
be a better predictor for heart disease in women than men.

There are conflicting reports as to the risk of obesity in
women, although these disagreements may be explained
by the findings that the pattern of fat distribution is more
relevant than the actual amount of excess fat. Women tend
to put on weight around the hips, so that, even if they are

obese, their hip measurement remains greater than their waist. Men tend to put on weight around the waist; all too often their belly protrudes well above the belt. It is the male pattern, whether in a man or a woman, that is associated with coronary disease. Abdominal obesity in a woman is associated with high blood pressure, high triglyceride and reduced HDL-C levels, and Type II diabetes—a cluster of conditions first given the attention grabbing label, the "Deadly Quartet," by the American physician Dr. Norman Kaplan.

There has been little investigation into the effects of such factors as family history or psychosocial interaction on women. Nevertheless, from the Framingham and other studies, the following trends have emerged. A family history of premature heart disease (a heart attack in a father or brother under the age of 55 years, or a mother or sister under the age of 65 years) carries an increased risk, as it does for men. However, there is some suggestion that the risk is stronger where the history is on the female side. Contrary to popular impression, the incidence of CHD is not higher in successful hard-driving career women. Rather it is greater in housewives, and also in those women who work in lower-paid jobs, in which they may have little or no control or authority.

There is not a great deal known about the effect of environmental stress on women compared with men. However, one intriguing research project has been carried out on a group of premenopausal macaque monkeys. The females of this species have a definite social status within their group and attempt to maintain or even improve that status (keeping up with or surpassing the Joneses, as it were). Over a ten-year period, batches of monkeys were exposed to stress by reducing their status and exchanging their dominant role for a more subdominant, submissive role. This change was achieved by putting them at the back of the line as they approached the water or food containers and depriving them of their rightful place to perch. All of the stressed females showed a marked drop in their HDL-C. Not only that, but they also developed severe coronary atherosclerosis. No such changes were observed in the non-stressed females. Further careful study revealed that the stressed females also showed an impairment of ovarian function, with the result that they had significantly lower levels of estrogen. This reduction in estrogen levels correlated closely with the fall in HDL-C and the appearance of severe coronary atherosclerosis.

We do know, however, that more than 60% of all women have one or more of the *known* major risk factors. There is every reason to believe that, having identified these individuals, we should be able to take preventive measures that will be every bit as successful as in men. Unfortunately, we do not seem to have been as able to convince women of this as we might like to think. For instance, over the past 25 years smoking among men has declined by about 50%, whereas in female teenagers it has increased. Obviously, when it comes to lung cancer and heart disease, we have been talking only to men. Contrary to the facts, women over 65 years continue to believe they are more likely to die from cancer than from a heart attack. The reality is that one in seven women between the ages of 45 and 64, and one in every three over the age of 65 have already developed evidence of coronary disease. We can only hope that future health promotion strategies will be designed with women in mind.

HEREDITY

As far as we know there is no specific gene for heart disease, although some families have a strong history of heart attacks. One possible explanation for this is the effect of family lifestyle. Children afflicted with parents who smoke are likely to take up smoking. Parents with no interest in physical recreation are unlikely to have sports-minded offspring. A teenager accustomed in the home or at school to a diet of fast food or one heavy in animal fat and dairy products has probably acquired a taste for these items and may find it very difficult to change in adult life. There is strong evidence for this viewpoint. Studies show that the spouses of patients with heart disease frequently go on to develop heart disease themselves. Since the chances that both had a genetic predisposition to heart disease are very remote, the most convincing explanation is that they developed the same disease because they shared the same high-risk environment.

The Ni-Hon-San (Nippon-Honolulu-San Francisco) study examined the incidence of heart attack deaths in Japanese living in Japan and those who had emigrated to Honolulu and San Francisco. As is typical for their country, those living in Japan had few heart attack deaths. Those who went to live in Honolulu had twice the heart attack death rate and those in San Francisco four times. There was no reason to believe that the three groups were genetically different. However, the lifestyle adopted by those living in San Francisco was thoroughly North American, whereas those living in Honolulu retained some of their cultural identity, including their dietary habits. Similar observations have been made on Jews emigrating to Westernized Israel, where heart disease is common, and from Yemen, where it is rare.

This is good news. We can prevent heart attacks by eliminating the modifiable risk factors. At the same time, it would be unfair not to consider the evidence of the influence of heredity. There may not be a "heart attack gene," but there is emerging proof that heredity does influence two of the major risk factors. For many years, it has been observed that high blood pressure tends to run in families, and a current theory has it that some of us inherit a tendency to develop this condition when exposed to certain environmental factors, such as psychological stress or a diet high in salt. It should be noted, however, that the adverse environmental factors must be present in order for the genetic predisposition to take effect. In other words, both seed and soil must come together.

In recent years, the most intriguing and exciting discoveries have been made in the area of high blood cholesterol, or hypercholesterolemia. In 1986, a major breakthrough was made by Drs. Brown and Goldstein, two American scientists, which won them the Nobel Prize. They established that the condition known as familial hypercholesterolemia was due to a genetic defect that led to the accumulation of high levels of LDL-C in the blood. Individuals with this condition invariably suffer a heart attack in their twenties or thirties, or in extreme cases in early childhood. It should be noted, however, that this disease exists in less than half of 1% of the population. But even here we are faced with the problem of seed and soil. In 1989, a unique study from the University of Utah traced the carriers of the gene for familial hypercholesterolemia through eight generations of a family that originated with a Mormon couple who were married in the 1790s. What emerged was a highly significant clue to our present-day coronary epidemic. Whereas those carriers living in the twentieth century either died from or developed manifestations of heart disease in their twenties or thirties, those who lived in the 1800s survived into their fifties, sixties, or even seventies. How could this be so? In the authors' words, "Male gene carriers born in this century tended to die at a younger age than male carriers of the same gene who were born in the nineteenth century.... It is likely that differences in diet or lifestyle may have affected disease severity in this family. The Utah pioneers were agrarian and physically active. Few members of this kindred living today have physically active occupations. Lifestyle and diet in the twentieth century gene carriers may account for the trend toward earlier death."

What seems to be emerging is that while some individuals inherit a susceptibility to atherosclerosis, they are probably balanced in the community by those at the other end of the spectrum who inherit a resistance to coronary disease. However, both groups make up only a small proportion of the population at large. Most of us are prone, not destined, to become victims of the so-called "good life" of the twentieth century.

HYPERTENSION (HIGH BLOOD PRESSURE)

What Is Blood Pressure?

Arterial blood pressure is expressed in two numbers, for example, 120/80 (stated as "one hundred and twenty over eighty"). The figures refer to millimeters of mercury (mm Hg). The first figure is the pressure in the arterial system when the heart is in the pumping phase of its cycle (systole) and is referred to as the systolic pressure. The second figure is the pressure when the heart is in the resting phase of its cycle (diastole) and is known as the diastolic pressure. The systolic pressure varies with the body's demand for oxygenated blood. For instance, during sleep when the muscles are relaxed, and all bodily functions are in the standby mode, the systolic pressure is low. During physical activity the working muscles burn oxygen at a faster rate and require an increased blood supply. The heart then steps up the speed and pressure with which it delivers blood into the arterial system. Thus the heart rate goes up, as does the systolic pressure. During a bout of all-out maximal exercise, the systolic blood pressure can increase to as much as 250 mm Hg. This is considered a normal response. The diastolic pressure, on the other hand, represents the constant background resting pressure in the arterial system. Even during extreme exercise, it normally does not increase by more than 20 mm Hg, for example, from 80 mm Hg to 100 mm Hg. Our blood pressure is clearly not a fixed measurement, as many mistakenly believe; it constantly fluctuates.

If this is the case, how can your physician make a diagnosis of high blood pressure? Well, strictly speaking the diagnosis should read *"resting* high blood pressure." This measurement is made when a person is relaxed. The instrument used, called a sphygmomanometer, consists of an inflatable cuff attached to a pressure-measuring system, usually a glass column of mercury. The cuff is placed around the upper arm, just above the elbow. In this position, it lies over an artery, called the brachial artery, which runs down the inside of the arm crossing the front of the elbow crease. In fact, if you straighten your elbow and place your fingertips over the inner half of the crease, you will probably feel the brachial artery pulsating.

To take the blood pressure, the cuff is inflated until the pulsation of the artery at the elbow can no longer be felt. The pressure at which the pulse is obliterated is the systolic pressure. The examiner continues to inflate the cuff another 10 or 15 mm Hg above this point, and then, listening with the stethoscope over the area where the pulse was felt, slowly reduces the pressure. Nothing will be heard until the level of systolic pressure, at which point the pulse will reappear and will be heard through the stethoscope. The cuff continues to be slowly deflated until the sounds disappear; this point is the diastolic pressure.

Resting blood pressure can vary considerably in healthy individuals, with systolic readings ranging from 90 to 140 mm Hg and diastolic from 60 to 90 mm Hg. Anxiety is a well-known blood pressure stimulator, and even the very act of having it taken by a doctor can raise it by 20 to 30 mm Hg (the so-called "white coat" syndrome). Other factors that may affect blood pressure, particularly in sensitive individuals, are painful stimuli, extreme cold, or even the discomfort of a full bladder. The subject, therefore, should be comfortable and at ease in order to obtain an accurate reading.

Of course, the sphygmomanometer must be accurate. The inflatable cuff should be the correct size to wrap around the arm comfortably. This is particularly important in the very fat arm, where an ill-fitting cuff can cause an inaccurate reading. The reading is generally taken with the patient either lying down or sitting comfortably, with the arm supported at approximately the same level as the heart. Two or more readings are usually taken two minutes apart. If the first two readings differ by more than 5 mm Hg, additional readings are taken and then averaged.

In recent years, physicians have taken to teaching their patients how to take their own blood pressure at home. By looking at the measurements taken at various times during the day over a period of weeks, they can get some idea of what the true resting blood pressure is. Another recent innovation is the ambulatory sphygmomanometer, which uses miniaturized digital equipment to measure, record, and store pressure readings every 15 to 30 minutes throughout the day and night. These can later be reproduced on a graph to show the daily fluctuations. Such devices are rather expensive and the original models had some teething problems. One early model made a soft but quite audible blowing noise as the cuff inflated and then slowly deflated. I recall giving one of these models to one of my patients to use over a 12-hour period. As it happened, he had to attend a protracted meeting of his board of directors the following day. Imagine his discomfort as on the hour, every hour, the directors were entertained by a short burst of soft but clearly audible snort-like sounds emanating from his person. Since they were too polite to enquire, and he too embarrassed to explain, the meeting must have been a memorable one. Thankfully, current models are inaudible.

Because diastolic pressure is less susceptible to transitory variations than systolic pressure, it is a better indicator of the day-to-day blood pressure level and is used frequently to define the presence or absence of hypertension. Why all this emphasis on the measurement of blood pressure? Because high blood pressure, sustained over a period of years, can have life-threatening consequences. It causes irreversible damage to the brain, heart, kidneys, blood vessels, and eyes. Unfortunately, it is not until the damage becomes obvious that symptoms appear and then it is often too late to do anything about it. Until then, high blood pressure causes no symptoms whatsoever, and its only sign is an elevated figure on the sphygmomanometer scale. It is now considered mandatory for everyone over the age of 30, and indeed even earlier for those with a family history of hypertension, to have their blood pressure checked annually.

What is normal blood pressure? A simple answer is the lower the better. It was thought that blood pressure increases with age, whence comes the outdated formula that a "normal" systolic pressure is "120 plus your age in years." Actually, only in urbanized industrialized societies does blood pressure increase with age. Primitive peoples living in their natural surroundings, such as certain groups of Australian Aborigines, the Inuit living in the Arctic, or the natives of New Guinea, have a low resting blood pressure throughout their adult years; it does not increase with age. In New Guinea and parts of South America where the incidence of stroke and hypertensive heart disease is extremely low, the diastolic blood pressure averages 60 mm Hg, approximately 20 points below the 80 mm Hg considered normal-average in our Western society.

Although elevated diastolic and systolic blood pressure usually go hand in hand, there is now strong evi-

CATEGORY	SYSTOLIC (mm Hg)		DIASTOLIC (mm Hg)
Optimal	<120	and	<80
Normal	<130	and	<85
High-Normal	130–139	or	85–89
Hypertension*			
Stage 1—borderline	140–159	or	90–99
Stage 2—moderate	160–179	or	100–109
Stage 3—severe	≥180	or	≥110
< Less than	≥ Equal or greater than	> Greater than	

* When systolic and diastolic blood pressures fall into different categories, the higher category should be used to classify the blood pressure status, e.g., 160/80 mm Hg should be classified as moderate hypertension, and 140/110 mm Hg as severe.

Figure 11: Classification of Blood Pressure Readings (Adapted from the guidelines of the National High Blood Pressure Education Program [1997])

dence that an elevated systolic blood pressure on its own can be a powerful predictor of stroke and heart disease. Furthermore, whereas it used to be thought that an isolated high blood pressure found on a casual reading could be ignored, it now appears that this can be a warning of the future development of permanent hypertension, and therefore periodic rechecks should be arranged. Figure 11 gives the currently accepted levels for hypertension.

Consequences of Hypertension

The major ill effects of hypertension are twofold: those directly due to the sustained pressure, and those due to associated coronary atherosclerosis. The constant high pressure in the arterial system throws an extra burden on the left ventricle of the heart, which compensates in the early stages by developing a thicker muscle wall, that is, it hypertrophies. Eventually, however, even the hypertrophied left ventricle is not up to the task, and it begins to weaken, dilate, and finally fail; it is unable to expel its entire contents with each beat, and blood begins to accumulate in the lungs. The patient notices increasing breathlessness, first on moderate then mild exertion, and finally even at rest. As the pressure backs up in the entire system, the right ventricle dilates, the water in the blood leaks out through the veins that return blood to the right side of the heart, and this excess fluid collects in the lower parts of the body, giving rise to swelling of the legs and feet. The patient is now in congestive heart failure. In addition to the direct effect on the heart, high pressures in the arteries to the brain, the kidneys, and the eyes can lead to strokes, kidney failure, and hemorrhages in the retina, respectively.

Hypertension is strongly associated with coronary atherosclerosis. Not only can it begin the atherosclerotic process by itself, it can also accelerate it in those who smoke or have high blood cholesterol. Hypertension places an extra burden on the vessel wall and damages the endothelium. Atheromas frequently occur where the vessels branch or bend and are thus directly exposed to the full force of the blood flow.

People with hypertension are two to three times more likely to sustain a heart attack than those with normal blood pressure, and this risk is higher in those over 60. The heart attack is more likely to be fatal in these people. Sudden cardiac death is also three to four times more common.

Although our primary interest in hypertension is as a risk factor for coronary heart disease, it is clearly also a disease in itself, from which as many as 50 million North Americans suffer.

Types of Hypertension
Doctors distinguish between secondary hypertension and essential hypertension. In secondary hypertension, blood pressure is elevated because one of the organs of the body

is diseased. The commonest cause is kidney disease. A diseased kidney releases a substance called renin into the bloodstream. Renin attempts to combat kidney failure by improving the organ's blood supply. It does this by increasing blood pressure, a scatter-gun approach at best. The kidney is helped only a little, whereas the cardiovascular system is seriously damaged. Secondary hypertension is relatively rare, comprising only about 5% of all cases of hypertension.

Essential hypertension occurs when there is no discernible causal disease; it is associated with 50% of all deaths in North America. It tends to run in families, with the child of a hypertensive parent more likely to develop it than one of a parent with normal blood pressure. If both parents are hypertensive, then the likelihood is even higher. Moreover, the more severely hypertensive the parents are, the more severe the hypertension in the offspring. Whether hypertension itself, or a susceptibility to developing hypertension in the presence of aggravating factors, is the inherited trait has not been established. What does seem to be certain is that there is a spectrum of environmental and acquired factors that, in certain individuals, enhance and accelerate the progress of the condition. These factors include age, body weight, diet, physical activity, and psychological stress.

Hypertension, Aging, and Obesity
In industrialized countries, people's blood pressure increases with aging, with about 50% of 65-year-olds being hypertensive. Since this is not seen in primitive societies, we can assume that hypertension is not necessarily a feature of growing old, but is a result of our modern lifestyle. One of the hallmarks of the affluent society is obesity. Surveys have shown that in the so-called advanced countries about one in five of us is overweight, and that one out of every three hypertensives is overweight. An

Australian study estimated that in 60% of male hypertensives under the age of 45, the aggravating factor was obesity. When obese hypertensives lose weight, their blood
pressure falls by about 2 mm Hg for every 2 pounds (1
kilogram) lost.

Hypertension and Diet

Various dietary constituents have been implicated in the
development of hypertension. The one you are probably
most familiar with is *salt*. There is a widespread impression that eating too much salt will lead to hypertension.
This theory was based on early work that showed that
populations with a very low salt intake had a low prevalence of hypertension. By the same token, communities
whose population ingested large quantities of salt had a
high prevalence of hypertension. Later studies, however,
thoroughly examined the relationship between salt intake
and blood pressure *within the same communities*. They did
not find the same association.

A large international investigation known as the
Intersalt Study has cast new light on the subject. Salt is a
combination of sodium and chloride, and, because
sodium is believed to cause the problem, this study determined salt intake by measuring the amount of sodium
excreted in the urine. The study, which involved 52 countries and some 10,000 subjects, found that in some of the
primitive communities, low sodium excretion in the urine
was associated with a low prevalence of hypertension.
However, in the majority of communities studied, the
relationship was not at all clear-cut.

What can we make of all of this? The current thinking
is that hypertensives are sensitive to salt. There is no
doubt that hypertensives who increase their salt intake
will increase their blood pressure, whereas hypertensives
who restrict salt intake will lower their blood pressure. The
problem is, you don't know whether you are salt-sensitive

or not until you discover you have hypertension. Reducing your salt intake at this stage is a bit like taking out health insurance after you get sick. So, since there is no benefit from a high salt intake, it can't do any harm and it may do a lot of good to reduce your salt intake while your blood pressure is still normal.

We should all limit our salt intake to six grams or less daily (six grams of salt contains about 2.4 grams of sodium). This amount includes salt added during cooking and at the table, and also the hidden salt found in processed and fast foods. Canned meats, canned soups, hot dogs, potato chips, salad dressings, and bottled sauces are a few examples of foods loaded with salt. If in doubt, always read the label and avoid processed foods that contain added salt.

If there is a debate about salt intake and hypertension, there is very little about alcohol consumption. Since the 1970s, a considerable body of evidence has accumulated to show a direct relationship between drinking habits and hypertension. Fewer than two drinks a day apparently have no effect, but thereafter the risk increases steadily. Those who regularly have two to four drinks a day have twice the incidence of hypertension; more than four drinks have three times the incidence. (A drink is generally defined as one containing 0.5 ounces [15 milliliters] of absolute alcohol. This is approximately the amount in a 1½-ounce [approximately a 50-milliliter] shot of 80 proof liquor, or 3 ounces [approximately 90 milliliters] of 20% fortified wine such as port or sherry, or 5 ounces [approximately 150 milliliters] of a 12% table wine, or one 12-ounce [355-milliliter] can of 4.5% beer.) Incidentally, you can't save your daily allowance up and drink it all in one session, although you might want to divide your weekly allowance into two or three portions and indulge on two or three occasions in the week to give your liver some time to recover! Most physicians now advise even their mildly hypertensive patients to restrict their alcohol intake, and the more severe hypertensives to abstain completely. The good news is that the effect of alcohol on hypertension is quickly reversible, and is seen as early as two weeks after cutting back.

Primitive societies in which salt intake is low also frequently have a high *potassium* intake from a diet rich in fresh fruit and vegetables. In some studies, the blood pressure of hypertensives who were given potassium supplement dropped 5 to 10 mm Hg. The current Canadian guidelines for the treatment of hypertensives therefore recommend that hypertensives, in addition to reducing their salt intake, also increase their dietary potassium intake to the maximum.

Calcium, like potassium, can also help to lower blood pressure. A number of large-scale nutritional studies have observed that hypertensives have a lower calcium intake. Experimental studies suggest that calcium supplements can decrease blood pressure in hypertensives. The recommended daily intake is 400–600 milligrams, and the most readily available source is milk, preferably in the form of skim milk, so as to avoid the saturated fat.

Whether a diet similar to that advocated for those with high blood cholesterol, that is, a diet low in saturated fat and high in polyunsaturated fat, can help hypertensives is still uncertain. Evidence in favor comes from the fact that vegetarians have a lower blood pressure than nonvegetarians. It seems unlikely that this is merely due to the lack of meat in their diet, but it could be the result of a low fat/high fiber content.

Hypertension and Stress
Although there is little direct evidence to associate hypertension with psychological stress, most physicians agree that many hypertensives are "race horse"-type people. They are often nervous and high-strung and tend to react

strongly to situations they perceive as threatening. It has been suggested that, at least in the early stages, the hypertensive state results from the body's "fight or flight" reaction, which releases adrenaline-like hormones into the bloodstream. A side effect of these hormones is an increase in blood pressure. If this occurs frequently over a long period of time, the body becomes accustomed to this higher blood pressure level and allows it to become permanent. We will discuss this again later in the context of exercise and its ability to reduce stress.

A number of stress-relieving strategies such as hypnosis, meditation, biofeedback, and muscular relaxation are now commonly used to relieve stress, but unfortunately few have been thoroughly evaluated. Studies indicate that biofeedback can result in some improvement, but the long-term effect is small. Greater improvements have been seen with a combination of these techniques.

Hypertension Drug Trials

A meta-analysis of 25 randomized trials, carried out over the past 30 years, which evaluated the effects of drug treatment in hypertensive persons (13 trials involving subjects over the age of 60 years and 12 involving those 60 and under) revealed that in the older patients, treatment reduced the death rate from stroke by 30%, and from heart attack by 25%. Both results were statistically significant. As for the trials in younger patients, these showed that treatment reduced death from stroke by a significant 40%, but deaths from heart attack only by 18%, a reduction which did not quite meet the 0.05 level of significance. However, if we add fatal and nonfatal heart attacks together, then the reduction amounts to 25%, and this is significant. Clearly, these randomized trials have established without doubt that treating elderly healthy hypertensives is highly effective. The slightly less dramatic results for fatal heart attack in younger hypertensives remains unexplained at this time, but this does not weaken the argument for timely intervention in all cases of elevated blood pressure.

Once hypertension is diagnosed, vigorous lifestyle modification is called for. In fact, the most recent (November 1997) guidelines used by the National High Blood Pressure Education Program recommend that patients suffering from mild hypertension (140–159/90–99 mm Hg) should try lifestyle changes before taking drugs. The strategy includes weight reduction for all patients who are more than 10% over their ideal body weight, a good aerobic exercise program, a low-salt, high-potassium-calcium diet, abstinence from smoking, and restricted alcohol intake. Even when drug therapy is required, it should be supplemented with advice about a healthy lifestyle. We now have adequate evidence that even a modest reduction in pressure of 5 to 10 mm Hg achieved by nonpharmacological means can ensure that the patient is controlled on minimal drug dosages, or may even eventually be able to stop medication altogether.

Lifestyle Changes for Reducing High Blood Pressure

- Lose weight if overweight
- Exercise regularly
- Limit alcohol intake to ≤1 oz/day
- Reduce sodium intake
- Maintain adequate dietary intake of potassium, calcium and magnesium
- Stop smoking
- Reduce fat intake

(Joint National Committee on the Treatment of Hypertension)

Table 1

DIABETES

The pancreas, a large gland situated in the abdominal cavity, secretes two hormones: glucagon and insulin. When blood sugar levels are low, glucagon stimulates the liver to release its stored glycogen into the blood in the form of glucose. When blood sugar levels are high, insulin facilitates the passage of glucose from the blood into the muscle cells, where it is burned for energy. In the condition known as diabetes, the pancreas is unable to secrete sufficient insulin, and glucose accumulates in the blood and spills out in the urine. The cells, deprived of the energy-rich fuel glucose, start to burn excessive amounts of fat or protein. This leads to the accumulation of toxic by-products in the blood, a condition that can cause coma and death. Diabetes was invariably fatal until the 1920s when two Toronto physicians, Drs. Banting and Best, isolated insulin from animal pancreas and successfully used it as an injectable replacement for human insulin.

Today, we recognize two main forms of diabetes, Type I and Type II. Type I is the classical form of the disease and the one most people are familiar with. Although it can appear at any age, it is generally first diagnosed in people under the age of 30. It is characterized by a total lack of insulin, requiring full replacement therapy by injection, and is often referred to as insulin-dependent diabetes. Type I diabetics are susceptible to a variety of complications including infections, problems with vision, nerve degeneration, and a special form of vascular disease involving the very small blood vessels (microvascular disease). Many or all of these can be largely avoided if the blood sugar is kept in control by a combination of diet and insulin.

Type II diabetes, or "late-onset" diabetes as it is also called, tends to develop in middle-aged or older individuals. There is growing awareness that this form of diabetes is a potent risk factor for coronary heart disease, increasing the risk twofold in men and four- to sixfold in women. What is even more alarming is that the condition is becoming very prevalent, almost an epidemic, and seems to be associated with our affluent modern lifestyle. As a consequence, it has attracted a good deal of research interest in recent years, with the emergence of the following facts. In Type II diabetics the pancreas secretes adequate amounts of insulin, but the body becomes increasingly incapable of utilizing it, i.e., it becomes "insulin-resistant." As a result, in an attempt to maintain normal blood sugar levels, the pancreas is stimulated to secrete more insulin. This works for a time, maybe even for as much as 10 or 15 years, but eventually the resistance to insulin becomes so strong that blood sugar levels begin to climb, and the patient presents with full-blown Type II diabetes. The fascinating part of the story, and one that has only begun to emerge, is that the increased risk for coronary heart disease develops, not as a result of the rise in blood sugar, but as a consequence of the years of abnormally high levels of blood insulin. In 1996, Jean-Pierre Després and his colleagues from Quebec City reported in the *New England Journal of Medicine* the results of their large-scale investigation of this problem. They collected blood samples for insulin levels from 2,000 healthy men aged 45 to 76 years, whom they then followed over a lengthy period in order to determine who would develop coronary heart disease. They discovered that the level of insulin at entry into the study was directly associated with the incidence of disease, those with the highest levels being most at risk. Further analysis of the data revealed that insulin remained a very strong predictor even when allowance was made for family history, hypertension, and blood cholesterol levels. Remember, when first seen, these men had not yet developed diabetes—their blood sugar levels were normal. Apparently, excess insulin leads to a cluster of coronary heart disease risk factors, for which an

American physician, Gerald Reaven, coined the term "Syndrome X" and which includes high blood pressure, elevation of the triglycerides and reduction in HDL-C levels (see Chapter 4), and an increased tendency for the blood to clot. One can readily see that Syndrome X sets the scene for heart disease.

But why do some of us become resistant to our insulin? There is no doubt that there are individuals in whom the tendency to develop Type II diabetes is inherited. Thus, if one or both parents have the condition, there is a high probability that it will emerge in the offspring. However, that is not the whole story. Certain racial groups also seem to be susceptible—but only when they are exposed to the full impact of our twentieth-century sedentary high-fat-diet lifestyle. Cases in point are the Pima Indians of New Mexico, Canada's Aboriginal population, and the native inhabitants of Polynesia. All have a considerably higher prevalence of diabetes than their Caucasian counterparts, all are relatively recent recruits to our slothful, overeating habits, and all have become subject to obesity. South Asians (natives of India, Pakistan, Bangladesh, and Sri Lanka) are another group who, when they adopt the Western lifestyle, tend to become obese, develop Type II diabetes, and are highly prone to coronary heart disease. In the opinion of some, obesity may be the trigger for the development of insulin resistance. This will be discussed later in this chapter.

We have seen that by the time blood sugar levels start to rise and Type II diabetes is diagnosed, the condition of hyperinsulinemia, or high blood levels of insulin, has been present for some time and has already accelerated the process of coronary atherosclerosis. How can we anticipate the diagnosis and take precautionary steps to avoid it? While it is possible to measure insulin levels, at the time of writing it still remains a research procedure and standardization of analysis techniques remains a problem.

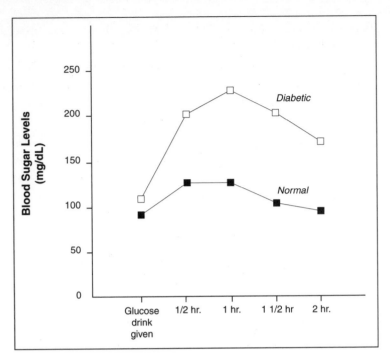

Figure 12: Glucose Tolerance Test
After taking a sugar drink, blood sugar should rise within half an hour, then return to pre-drink level within one and a half to two hours. In diabetics, the initial rise is higher and the blood sugar level has not returned to normal after one and a half to two hours. This test can yield an abnormal result *before* **the onset of diabetic symptoms, a condition known as chemical or latent diabetes.**

Eventually measurement of fasting insulin levels will become good practice in the early detection of type II diabetes and even coronary artery disease. In the meantime, there is a test we can use which can help. It is called a *glucose tolerance test*. First, the blood glucose is measured after fasting overnight. The patient then drinks a glucose solution, after which blood samples are taken every half hour for at least two hours, and blood glucose levels measured each time. Blood glucose will rise quickly after the drink, but if insulin sensitivity is normal it will have returned to resting levels by the end of the two hours. If, on the other hand, it fails to do so, one can assume that there is some degree of insulin resistance and that the body is likely producing excessive amounts of insulin in order to compensate for this (Figure 12). This condition is referred to as "glucose intolerance," and affects some 20% of individuals middle-aged and older. Glucose intolerance is a precursor of Type II diabetes. Thus, if there is a family history of Type II diabetes, it is wise to have your doctor arrange for a glucose tolerance test annually after you reach the age of 40.

How does one treat Type II diabetes—or for that matter glucose intolerance? The two mainstays of treatment are diet and exercise. Some patients will require the addition of a daily tablet to regulate blood glucose (insulin injections are rarely required), hence the other name for Type II diabetes, non-insulin-dependent diabetes (NIDD).

CIGARETTE SMOKING

Everyone is now aware of the connection between cigarette smoking and lung cancer. How many also realize that the smoker is three to four times more likely to experience a heart attack than the nonsmoker, and that the attack is more likely to be fatal? The risk increases proportionally with the number of cigarettes smoked and is particularly high in those under the age of 50. The risk of *sudden cardiac death* increases more than tenfold in men and fivefold in women who smoke.

According to the American Academy of Pediatrics, more than 3,000 children and teenagers in the United States start to smoke each day. Furthermore, while there has been a sharp decline in the number of men in the 20-to-25 age bracket who start the smoking habit, there has been a sharp increase in new women smokers in the same age bracket. If the trend continues, soon we can expect that more women than men will smoke. The British medical authorities have come up with the sobering statistic that of every thousand young adults who smoke, 250 will die from a smoking-related disease. Although there is growing opposition in the West to tobacco advertising and its targeting of the young, the developing countries have yet to take a similar stance; unless they do, they will face a similar epidemic of lung cancer and heart disease. The tobacco industry is now targeting the developing countries, and apparently with considerable success. Will these nations eventually have to face a problem of equal magnitude?

Tobacco smoke contains more than 2,000 known substances, including nicotine, carbon monoxide, nitrogen dioxide, benzine, formaldehyde, and hydrogen cyanide. Many of these compounds are capable of damaging the endothelial lining of the coronary arteries and thereby provoking atherosclerosis. Probably the two major harmful compounds are nicotine and carbon monoxide. The nicotine in cigarette smoke is highly addictive. It is released into the bloodstream within seven seconds of inhaling the smoke and almost immediately triggers the release of adrenaline and a related substance called noradrenaline. These two hormones, which are produced by the adrenals, two small glands just above the kidney, prepare the body for "fight or flight." As a result, blood pressure rises and heart rate goes up, increasing the heart muscle's requirements for oxygen. Unfortunately, however, this demand is thwarted by the action of the other substance in tobacco smoke, carbon monoxide, which is also the principal poisonous ingredient in car exhaust fumes. In large doses, carbon monoxide kills by displacing all the oxygen in the red blood cells. Actually, hemoglobin, the protein in the red cell that carries oxygen, *prefers* carbon monoxide and, given the choice, is 200 times more likely to pick it up than oxygen. You can see the paradox. Nicotine increases the heart muscle's oxygen requirements, and carbon monoxide makes sure that those requirements are not met.

If the coronary arteries are already narrowed and the blood supply to the heart limited as a result of atherosclerosis, smoking makes matters worse. Anginal sufferers who smoke experience pain at a much lower level of exertion than nonsmokers. Even in the absence of coronary atherosclerosis, heavy smoking may cause heart attacks. There are reports of young heavy-smoking adults who have suffered a heart attack and yet on subsequent investigation are found to have normal coronary arteries. The mechanism is a shutdown of the coronary artery due to a spasm provoked by exposure to nicotine. In susceptible individuals, nicotine can cause life-threatening irregularities of the heartbeat. Sudden cardiac death is thereby probably another hazard for smokers. A number of investigators have also established that smokers have "sticky" blood and are liable to develop clots in their arteries, particularly the coronary vessels or the vessels in the leg. Finally, it has been noted that habitual smokers have lower levels of the protective HDL-C. Since a high HDL-C is felt to be one of the major mechanisms that protects young women from coronary disease, this might explain why women who smoke seem to have lost that protection.

It is extremely hard for most people to give up smoking. As an ex-smoker myself, I sympathize with anyone trying to quit. Experts in the field have said that in some ways addiction to cigarettes is as strong as, if not stronger than, addiction to heroin. The acute physical withdrawal symptoms may not be so severe, but apparently the craving is never quite extinguished. Many individuals who stopped smoking for 20 or even 30 years have started again after a few casual cigarettes. After 30 years of working with cardiac patients at the Toronto Centre, we are now experiencing this phenomenon. Admittedly the numbers are small, but some people who were enrolled in our program in the late 1960s, and who stopped smoking after their heart attack, have started again after 20 years. To be hon-

est, I have to say that if somebody were to offer me a perfectly safe cigarette now (and such a cigarette is nowhere
in sight), even 30 years after quitting I would be tempted
to start smoking again!

There is no safe alternative to quitting. Low-tar, low-
nicotine filter cigarettes have been found to be just as dangerous as their predecessors, since habitual smokers will
continue to get their boost of nicotine by taking deeper,
more frequent puffs and smoking the cigarette right down
to its filter. Pipe and cigar smokers are at slightly less risk
than those who smoke cigarettes, but this is apparently not
the case for former cigarette smokers. Having once
learned to inhale from a cigarette, smokers invariably
apply the same practice to a pipe or cigar.

How quickly after you quit can you expect to reduce
your risk for a heart attack? Nicotine is quickly cleared
from the body (which is why you experience early withdrawal symptoms). Carbon monoxide takes about 24 hours
to clear, but by then its ill effects will have gone. One to two
weeks after stopping, the risk starts to decrease, and a number of studies have demonstrated that it reaches almost the
level of a nonsmoker at the end of one to two years.

Danger to Nonsmokers
In recent years, there has been increasing recognition of the
dangers to nonsmokers of sidestream smoke, that is, the
smoke that escapes into the air from the burning end of the
cigarette for all to inhale, smokers and nonsmokers alike.
In fact, this danger has been the major impetus for the
banning of smoking in public places. Actually, sidestream
smoke contains a higher concentration of nicotine, carbon
monoxide, and other pollutants than exhaled (mainstream) smoke. Obviously, the danger to the nonsmoker
is greater in confined areas. A Scottish study looked at the
effect on a nonsmoker living with a spouse who smoked.
More than 15,000 men and women were followed up for

an average of 11.5 years. The nonsmoking spouses of smokers had two and a half times the incidence of lung cancer and twice the incidence of heart disease compared with the nonsmoking spouses of nonsmokers. Further American and British studies have confirmed that exposure to second-hand smoke can increase the risk of heart attack by 20%–30%.

There has been a recent resurgence in the use of a very old form of tobacco, snuff. Oral snuff is now packed in small bags that are held between the gum and cheek. With the help of heavy promotion by the tobacco industry, and the example set by the "boys of summer," the baseball players, the use of oral snuff in the United States has increased 15-fold since 1970, largely in 17- to 19-year-old young men. Oral snuff, since it delivers nicotine to the bloodstream, albeit not so quickly as inhaled cigarette smoke, is nevertheless addictive and frequently leads to cigarette smoking itself. Apart from that, this form of tobacco causes cancer of the mouth, throat, and stomach. In 1990, Britain banned the sale of oral snuff, and similar bans are also in force in Israel, New Zealand, Hong Kong, Singapore, and Japan. How long will it take for North America to follow suit?

Years ago, more than I care to remember, when I first started talking to post–heart attack patients, I was often asked "How come my grandfather started to roll his own when he was 12 years old and smoked until he was 90, and he never had a heart attack or lung cancer?" In those days I would answer condescendingly, "Well, your grandfather isn't you, and you are not your grandfather. You are the one who has had the heart attack, and your grandfather was one in a million"—or words to that effect. In retrospect, I realize I probably antagonized the questioners and did nothing to convince them of the dangers of smoking. Now that I am older and, I hope, wiser, I would answer the question differently. I would admit that we don't have a full explanation for Grandfather's apparent immunity from heart disease (I can't speak for cancer), but the question is being researched fully and already there are some interesting data.

Take the situation in Japan. The incidence of coronary disease there is among the lowest in the world. On my first visit to that country, I was staggered to see how many men smoked. Subsequent visits confirmed this impression, and ultimately I was not surprised to learn that the Japanese consumption of cigarettes per capita is one of the highest in the world; and yet the incidence of CHD is very low. However, if we pick out the countries with a high incidence of heart disease, such as the United States, the United Kingdom, Europe, and Australia, smoking emerges as a risk factor.

The implication is that smoking often requires the presence of some other coronary risk factor, either known or unknown. Laboratory experimental evidence indicates that one of the major constituents of tobacco smoke, carbon monoxide, will damage the endothelial lining of the coronary artery, but in the absence of high blood cholesterol levels, the atherosclerotic plaque does not form. This would explain why smoking is strongly associated with increasing atherosclerosis in Western countries, where the average blood cholesterol levels are high, as opposed to Japan, where the average blood cholesterol levels are extremely low. Further evidence for the argument that smoking provokes coronary risk factors is found in the fact that hypertensives who smoke are five times more likely to go on to develop an extremely severe and often fatal form of the disease called malignant hypertension. Also, as we have seen, women smokers on the birth control pill incur a risk of heart disease that is 20 times as high as that faced by nonsmokers. Of course, none of this should be taken as a mandate for people without other risk factors to smoke. After all, the Japanese do suffer from lung cancer and have a very high incidence of stroke. Finally, if you live in the coronary-prone West, you might as well accept that the smoking habit puts you in double jeopardy.

Quitting Smoking

The acute symptoms of nicotine withdrawal last for about two weeks and, while not disabling, they are certainly not pleasant. They include irritability, insomnia, depression, and inability to concentrate. The more cigarettes smoked, the worse the symptoms. All strategies to stop smoking are designed to reduce the discomfort of nicotine withdrawal and then modify subsequent behavior so as to prevent a return to smoking.

It goes without saying that those people who are the most highly motivated to give up the habit are the most likely to succeed. One way to sharpen motivation is to spend a week or two writing down all the reasons to stop, to review the list daily, and then to inform family, relatives, and friends of the intention to stop—in short, to make it a big event.

Groups led by professional counsellors have about a 35% greater success rate over a 12-month follow-up period than those who tried to stop on their own. Once the program starts, the first aim is to reduce the effects of nicotine withdrawal. One way to do this is to use nicotine-replacement therapy, utilizing gum, patch, or spray. Used by motivated people in conjunction with group education and counselling, it has a reported success rate greater than 80%. In less-motivated individuals, or taken casually and without accompanying support, its results have not been quite so successful. Acupuncture was widely acclaimed for a time, but the initial enthusiasm for this approach seems to have abated. Hypnosis is still popular, and in the early days of the Toronto Centre's cardiac program, we used it as an adjunct to exercise in postcoronary patients. It was reasonably successful in improving morale and self-confidence in certain patients, but the numbers were too small for us to judge its benefit in smoking cessation.

Some organized programs have a preparatory run-in period, during which the subject is exposed to techniques that attempt to break the association between nicotine and a pleasurable sensation. Forcing oneself to smoke a number of cigarettes in rapid succession and rinsing the mouth with solutions that give a bad taste to the smoke are just two of the methods used. Again, the results have not been subjected to scientific trial, but patients who have attended these programs report some success. A gradual reduction in the daily consumption of cigarettes to soften the shock of the eventual cessation is another reasonable approach, and there is a small "computer" device on the market that signals when it is time for a smoke, the signals becoming less frequent over a two- to three-week period.

Once having stopped for two to four weeks, the individual faces the problem of relapse. During this stage the ex-smoker will inevitably begin to rationalize the need to start again. Weight gain is probably one of the most common reasons given, even though it rarely reaches a level that constitutes a health hazard. An appropriate diet and a suitable exercise program can help avoid this consequence. A system of reward also helps. A good move is to put the money saved by not smoking in a separate bank account, and every six months spend some or all of it on some pleasurable luxury. Constantly reminding oneself of the health benefits of giving up can be a great incentive, as is the fact that food tastes better, clothes don't smell, and one is free from the never-ending fear of running out of cigarettes.

I believe that once a person makes up his or her mind to quit, a regular program of physical activity can be of the greatest help. Each workout releases into the bloodstream a charge of adrenaline, which can be a good substitute for nicotine. The steady improvement of fitness is tangible evidence of physical benefit, and the tendency to put on weight is prevented. This approach worked well for me, as well as for many of my cardiac patients.

STRESS

When we asked patients referred to the Toronto Centre's cardiac program in the 1970s what they believed caused their heart attack, six out of ten put stress at the top of their list. After attending for three months, they attached more importance to smoking, lack of exercise, and diet. Invariably, however, stress was still mentioned as an important factor. In the past three or four years, new patients have had a greater tendency to put diet on top, but stress is still considered important. Many people think that the stress of modern living is one of the main causes of our twentieth-century heart attack epidemic. Part of the reason we blame stress is that it is easier than blaming our own eating or smoking habits. Stress is something that our boss or the government or society has laid on us. It is beyond our control.

But although we all feel that stress must be a factor in coronary disease, few studies have addressed it. Part of the reason is that we do not have a satisfactory method to measure stress. In fact, there is no universally accepted definition of stress. The term was first popularized by Dr. Hans Selye, who borrowed the word from physics. Dr. Selye used it to describe the body's responses to a variety of harmful physical stimuli, such as extreme cold or chronic sleep deprivation. These bodily responses are primitive and date back to a period early in our evolution when the environment was hostile but relatively simple. Faced with danger, primitive people usually had only two courses: stand and fight, or turn and run. Either way, excessive muscular activity was called for, and the body responded by releasing hormones (adrenaline and noradrenaline) into the bloodstream, which set the stage for action. These hormones increase the heart rate and blood pressure, thus ensuring a rapid delivery of oxygenated blood to the muscles. At the same time, they free up the stored fat and sugar from the fat depots and the liver, raising blood fat and blood sugar levels to make them readily available to the muscles for fuel. Breathing is quickened to augment oxygen uptake. Finally, and just in case the action results in cuts or bruises, the blood becomes "stickier" and will clot more easily to staunch any bleeding. The body is now like a tightly wound spring, straining to uncoil. This condition has been referred to as the "fight or flight" response (Figure 13). If physical action takes place, then the spring unwinds. Heart rate, blood pressure, blood levels of fat, sugar, and clotting substance all return to normal.

Let us apply this to modern life, where things are not so simple. Innumerable situations in our complex urban civilization pose a real or perceived threat to our peace of mind. Although the environment has changed, however, our response has not. It is still as primitive as ever. We are all familiar with the quickened heartbeat and breathing and the flushed face that accompany an argument or a feeling of panic. Rarely, however, is physical action an appropriate response. We cannot settle our day-to-day conflicts by fighting, or by running away. Nowadays, we rarely face physical dangers. Most of our problems are associated with personal finances, difficulties on the job, or interpersonal relations. Generally, these are solved with varying degrees of ease and form the background of normal living. This general level of tension is what Dr. Selye referred to as eustress, or good stress. Without it, life would be dull, bland, and uninteresting. There is evidence that in the total absence of eustress, we would develop severe physical and psychological derangements. As a matter of fact, many of us crave a degree of potentially harmful physical

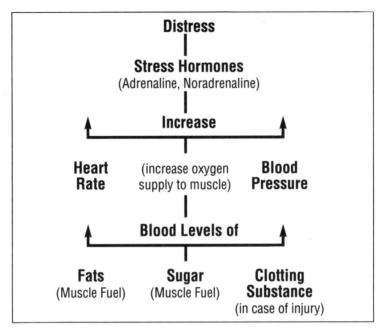

Figure 13: Fight or Flight Response

stress. Why else do so many take part in dangerous sports such as mountaineering, climbing, and automobile and motorcycle racing?

When does eustress become distress? Essentially, when we are faced with a threat to our well-being that we cannot solve. We are unable to cope. The spring is coiled, but there is no release. We are tense and anxious; our blood pressure, blood fat, and blood sugar levels are raised, and our blood is sticky and will clot easily. If this state of affairs persists in an individual who already suffers from narrowed atherosclerotic coronary arteries, then it requires no great stretch of the imagination to recognize the potential for a clot forming within one of those arteries, causing a heart attack.

This scenario is persuasive, and answers some of the apparent inconsistencies that arise from attributing the coronary epidemic entirely to a diet high in animal fat. For example, examination of the London Hospital's autopsy records for the period 1901 to 1952 reveals that over that period of time there had been no change in the extent of atherosclerosis in the coronary arteries. This evidence would suggest that our grandparents had just as much coronary disease as we have. On the other hand, from the 1920s on, there was a steady increase in the number of old scars detected in the heart muscle, a measure of the number of heart attacks that occurred during life. This finding would suggest that the change that occurred in the 1920s was not an increase in the extent of coronary atherosclerosis but some factor that increased intracoronary blood clotting. We shall look at this whole topic again when we deal with the relationship of physical activity to heart disease.

Establishing the mechanism by which stress can cause a heart attack still doesn't help us too much when it comes to identifying or quantifying it. What is stressful for one individual is pleasurable to another. Some of us delight in long hours and working to deadlines; others feel threatened and can cope only with the help of excessive alcohol, tobacco, or food. Contrary to popular opinion, many studies have been unable to find an increase in heart disease in high-level executives. Some 270,000 employees of the Bell Telephone Company were observed over a five-year period. Senior executives with heavy responsibility were actually found to have a lower incidence of heart attacks. Other studies in Sweden and Israel reached similar conclusions.

It is obviously very difficult to identify objectively a set of environmental circumstances everyone will find stressful. Nevertheless, efforts have been made to do just that. Probably one of the most widely used, the Social Readjustment Rating Scale, is based on the assumption that major life changes are themselves a source of stress because the adjustment they require imposes a psychological and physiological burden. If the adjustment period is lengthy, or a multiplicity of changes occurs over a given period, usually one or two years, then the constant state of arousal ultimately breaks down the body's defenses and results in illness. The scale consists of 43 items, including "death of spouse," "divorce," "marital separation," "fired from work." While the authors of the scale found that retrospectively it correlated well with the incidence of heart attacks and sudden death, other investigators using prospective studies were unable to show any relationship between the scores and subsequent cardiovascular events. Another school of thought places less importance on the relatively infrequent major events in one's life and maintains that stress results from the accumulation of frequent daily irritants and events that force one through constant adjustment and adaptation. A list of common, minor irritants has been developed into the 117-item Hassle Scale, and initial work suggests that it might be a better predictor of stress-related illnesses than the major-life-events approach.

Based on their studies, Drs. Mayer Friedman and Ray Rosenman have come up with a description of the coronary-prone personality. These aggressive achievers are ambitious and constantly attempt to accomplish more and more in less and less time. As soon as a goal is attained, they immediately set another, higher than the last. Characteristically, they are very time-conscious (woe betide you if you are late for an appointment with one), impatient (they rarely let the other person finish a sentence), speak in short explosive sentences, and are highly competitive. In short, they could be the role model for a highly successful businessperson. These individuals are classified as being personality Type A. In contrast, Type B personalities are described as less competitive, less time-conscious, more interested in cultural and artistic rather than business values, patient and relaxed. Type As, according to the theory, over-react to all challenges and are more susceptible to coronary disease.

This theory gained much support and a large following in the 1970s. Then in 1981 one of the first dissenting reports appeared. In a group of 189 heart attack survivors, X-rays of the coronary arteries (coronary angiography) failed to show any association between Type A personality and the extent or degree of coronary atherosclerosis. When these patients were followed up after discharge from the hospital, more fatal recurrent heart attacks occurred in Type Bs than in Type As. From then on, the case against the existence of a coronary-prone personality became even stronger. A complete review of all the data shows that whereas prior to 1977 the evidence was favorable, since then large well-designed studies have increasingly diminished the importance of Type A behavior.

Nevertheless, now that the initial fervor has passed, it may still be profitable to look more closely at the concept, since it still retains some tantalizingly attractive aspects. For instance, it has been suggested that a hostile attitude is the major component in a Type A personality that predicts future coronary events, and that current methods of screening are not sensitive enough to detect this hostility. Alternatively, if Type A behavior is harmful because it involves a constant readiness for "fight or flight," then measurement of heart rate, blood pressure, and blood levels of stress hormones, cholesterol, and sugar in response to a standard stressful task, such as solving a difficult mathematical problem in front of onlookers, would permit a more accurate and objective selection of the true hyperreactors than the presently used psychological interview and personality questionnaire.

Although the jury is still out, stress management has become one of the leading growth industries of our day. Books, clinics, counsellors, and audiovisual instruction kits abound. In the early days of the Toronto program we used hypnosis, and later yoga, to improve mood. Both methods had some success, but in our experience neither is as effective as a good exercise training program. In fact, for most of us, I would have to put exercise at the top of my list as the easiest, most readily available and successful method of coping with day-to-day stressful situations.

OBESITY

The word obese comes from the Latin *obesus*, meaning "that has eaten himself to fat." There couldn't be a better description of what has been identified as one of the most important public health problems for our times. The obese are prone to a list of ailments, including heart disease, high blood pressure, Type II diabetes, gall bladder disease, cancer of the bowel and prostate in men, cancer of the breast and uterus in women, osteoarthritis of weight-bearing joints, bronchitis and asthma, accidents, etc.; the long list is frightening. Much of what we know about the dangers of being overweight has been gained from the massive amount of information gathered by the insurance industry. From their data, we have been able to formulate tables that relate body weight to height and also identify a "desirable" weight, above which there is an increased risk of illness and premature death. The most commonly used table in North America is the one drawn up by the Metropolitan Life Insurance Company, 1983 version. You can roughly calculate your ideal weight, if you are of medium frame, from the following: men—106 pounds (48 kilograms) for the first 5 feet (1.5 meters), and 6 pounds (2.7 kilograms) for each additional inch (2.5 centimeters); women—100 pounds (45 kilograms) for the first 5 feet (1.5 meters), and 5 pounds (2.3 kilograms) for each additional inch (2.5 centimeters). If you are 20% above ideal weight, this is defined as being overweight; 30% above ideal is considered obese.

Lean Body Mass and Percentage Body Fat

You will note that the definition of the Latin word *obesus* used the word fat, and with good reason. When you step on the scales, you get a measurement of your overall body weight, which includes the weight of your fat mass *and* your nonfat mass. Your nonfat mass, referred to by scientists as your lean body mass, is the total weight of your muscle and bone tissue. Lean body mass usually varies with height, which explains why height and weight are linked in the Metropolitan Life tables. In healthy men, the fat mass is said to be 15% to 20% of the total body weight, and in healthy women 25% to 30% of the total. Excess weight is considered to be due entirely to fat mass. It is this excess fat mass that leads to the health problems associated with being overweight. Whereas the weight tables are a satisfactory guide for most of us, there are exceptions. For example, an ardent weight lifter or body-builder will have excessive musculature and a dispropor-tionately large lean mass. On the other hand, a very elderly person, in whom lack of any physical activity often leads to muscle wasting, will have disproportion-ately large fat mass.

If fat content is what we are interested in, why don't we measure it directly? The simple answer is that we do, but it's not as easy as it sounds. The most accurate method we have can be used only in a properly equipped exercise laboratory. It is known as underwater, or hydrostatic, weighing. First, you are weighed on standard scales on dry land. Then, sitting in a sling or suspended chair, you are totally submerged in a tank of water and weighed again. Since fat weighs less than water, you will weigh less sub-merged. The underwater weight is then subtracted from the dry weight and the result incorporated into a series of complex equations from which we derive a value for per-centage of body fat.

An easier and more frequently used method is the measurement of skinfolds. The test is carried out by pinching a fold of skin and its underlying fat between the finger and thumb and measuring its thickness with a pair of specially designed calipers. This is done at several locations on the body. The measurements are generally combined in a mathematical equation that gives a predicted value for total body fat. This method is most frequently used by exercise physiologists, and in the hands of someone experienced in the use of the caliper and the correct choice of skinfold sites, it correlates closely with the results of underwater weighing.

You can obtain a reasonable estimate of your own fat layer by pinching a transverse fold of skin and fat over your abdomen, one inch (2.5 centimeters) below your navel. Ideally, this fold should be no more than half an inch (1 centimeter). The fat fold over the back of your upper arm, halfway between your shoulder and elbow, should be no more than one inch (2.5 centimeters) (one and a half inches or 3.5 centimeters in women).

Body Mass Index
The most universal method of measuring body fat is the Quatelet index, or the Body Mass Index (BMI). This method has been adopted by Health and Welfare Canada and many other health professionals and government agencies throughout the world. The BMI is the figure obtained by formula from the body weight and the height. Its purpose is to minimize the effect of height-related tissue (lean body mass). For ease of use, a "nomogram" (graph) has been developed that enables you to plot your BMI from your height and your weight and is shown on the next page (Figure 14).

A BMI between 20 and 25 is considered to be desirable, since it is associated with the lowest risk of illness. A value of 25 to 30 is regarded as overweight. It represents a moderate degree of obesity and can be associated with some

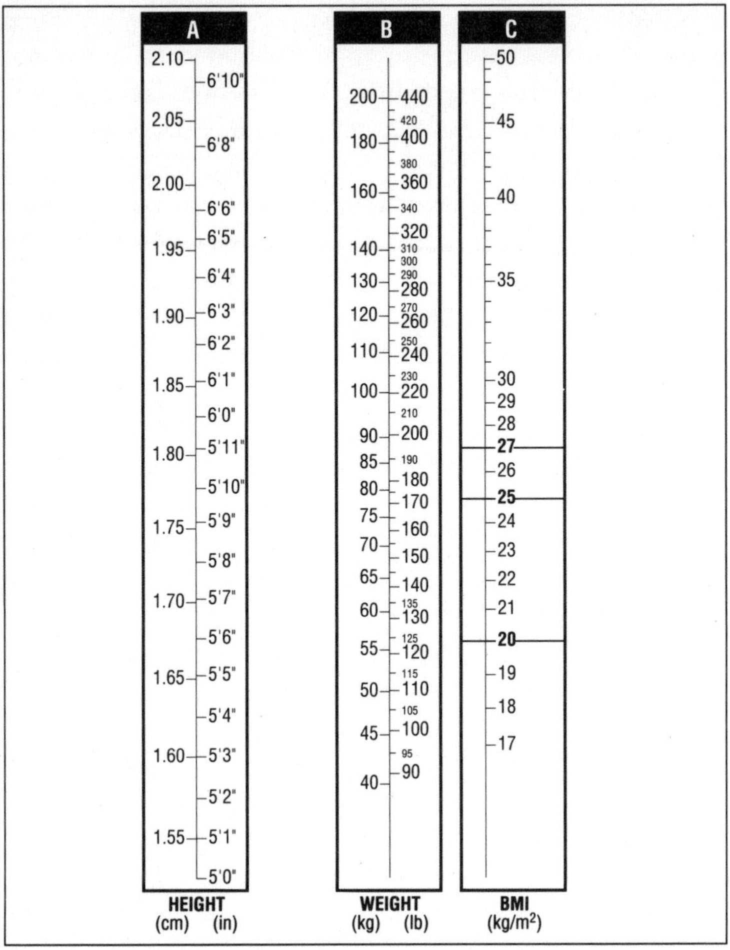

A	B	C
HEIGHT (cm) (in)	WEIGHT (kg) (lb)	BMI (kg/m²)

Figure 14: Body Mass Index (BMI)

To determine your body mass index: (1) Mark an x at your height on scale A; (2) Mark an x at your weight on scale B; (3) Use a ruler to extend a straight line drawn through your height and weight to intersect with scale C. Wherever the line meets scale C is your BMI.

A BMI in the range of 20-25 is generally healthy.

A BMI in the range of 25-27, though acceptable, should alert you to the possibility of developing health problems.

A BMI greater than 27 indicates the possibility of developing health problems, such as high blood pressure, diabetes, heart disease.

Note: BMI should not be used with children and those under 20 years, with adults over 65, with pregnant and lactating women, or with muscular individuals.

health risks. A BMI of 30 or higher is inevitably due to obesity and is associated with a higher death rate from the diseases listed above. Using this classification, figures from North America, Australia, the United Kingdom, and Europe show that about 35% of men and 25% of women fall in the category of moderately obese and a further 6% of men and 8% of women are markedly obese. It would seem that almost half the adult population of the industrialized world is too fat.

Body Fat Distribution
Jean Vague was a Professor of Medicine in Marseilles, France, in the 1940s. He had a particular interest in obesity and noted that his overweight patients were prone to a multitude of ills, including diabetes, atherosclerosis and arthritis. Of greater importance, however, was his observation that there were two types of fat distribution in his obese patients. In the male type the fat was deposited around the trunk (truncal, or android obesity) and in the female type, the excess fat was stored primarily around hips and thighs (female, or gynoid obesity). The distinction was important, because, as Professor Vague pointed out, it was only the truncal obesity, whether present in a man or a woman, that was associated with major health problems. A number of large-scale studies have since confirmed this finding, and it is now generally accepted that the quantity of fat may not be as important as where it is situated (Figure 15).

THE DEADLY QUARTET

Truncal obesity is a visible sign of excess fat in the abdominal cavity, where it surrounds and infiltrates the walls of the intestines. Indeed, for every pound of visible fat around the waist, there is another pound of invisible fat

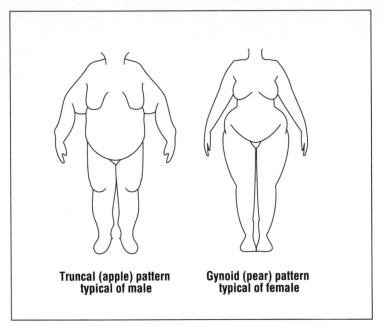

**Truncal (apple) pattern
typical of male**   **Gynoid (pear) pattern
typical of female**

Figure 15: Patterns of Obesity

enveloping the gut. We now know that this additional load of fatty tissue alters the body's chemical system in such a way as to dramatically affect the way it metabolizes both sugar and fat. This chain of events has been termed, by the American physician Dr. Norman Kaplan, the Deadly Quartet (Figure 16). Truncal obesity leads to insulin resistance, which in turn leads to excessive levels of blood insulin, and because insulin is a salt-retaining hormone, salt levels rise and this causes hypertension. As resistance to insulin increases, its effectiveness wanes, blood sugars rise, Type II diabetes develops, and as a side effect of this there is a derangement of fat metabolism characterized by elevated blood triglycerides and reduced levels of "good" cholesterol. As you will note, the Deadly Quartet and Syndrome X (page 190) are two attention-getting terms for the same chain of events, although the latter emphasizes the role of central obesity as the first link in the chain.

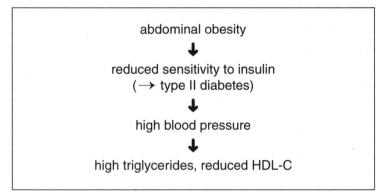

Figure 16: The Deadly Quartet

Whichever term you prefer to use, you can readily say that both set the scene for the development of coronary heart disease—and both are brought about largely as a result of eating too much and exercising too little!

Causes of Obesity

The children of obese parents often grow up to be obese themselves. Surveys show that when both parents are fat, three-quarters of their children will be obese; when both are thin, only 9% will be fat. This connection has led to the speculation that obesity is an inherited trait, and to the all-too-familiar argument between heredity and environment, or nature and nurture. Evidence in favor of heredity comes from studies of adopted children, who tend to take after their natural rather than their adoptive parents insofar as body build is concerned. By the same token, identical and non-identical twins strongly resemble one another in height, body weight, and fat distribution, regardless of whether they were raised together or apart.

A genetic factor does seem to contribute to obesity. Nevertheless, it is obvious that eating too much and exercising too little will make you fat whether you have inherited the tendency to become so or not. It may be easier to put on weight and more difficult to lose it if it is a family trait, but without the imbalance between high-calorie input and low-calorie burn, fat cannot accumulate.

The manner in which fat is stored also throws some light on the problem. The fat storage depots consist of collections of fat cells. We can increase the amount of fat in these depots in only two ways: the fat cells can increase in size (fat cell hypertrophy), or the fat cells can increase in number (fat cell proliferation). Proliferation is very active in the fetus during the last three months of pregnancy and the first year of life, after which it continues at a slower rate up until age ten or so, and then in spurts during growth periods of adolescence. There is generally little further increase during adulthood, although it can occur if the caloric intake is high and energy output low. Fat cell hypertrophy occurs in much the same manner, until by adulthood a maximum size has been reached. This size cannot be exceeded. One final point: *Once fat cells are added, they cannot be lost.* Therefore, weight reduction is achieved by *reduction in the size, not the number, of fat cells.* Because the number of cells remains the same, there is always the potential for them to pick up more fat, which explains why it is so easy to put on weight again after reducing.

Since cell proliferation is so active during early life, dietary and exercise habits adopted during this period have far-reaching consequences. Even the mother-to-be's pattern of weight gain during the final three months of pregnancy may be of considerable importance. For instance, we know that pregnant women who gain excessive weight during the final trimester frequently produce babies with a higher percentage of body fat than those in whom the mother's weight gain was within desirable limits. Furthermore, if children are exposed to a sensible program of nutrition and regular physical activity, they are less likely to enter their adult years with an excess number of fat cells and to face a lifelong battle with obesity.

Surveys show that 80% of fat children grow up to be fat adults. As for adults, increase in body weight first results in the fat cells taking up more fat. Once they have taken on as much as their size will allow, additional fat can be stored only by manufacturing more fat cells. *This occurs when the degree of obesity exceeds 30% of the desirable weight.* Since weight reduction cannot be achieved by reducing the numbers of cells, the only alternative is shrinking the cells to a size less than that which has been genetically determined. This throws an extra burden on the body and makes weight reduction all the more difficult.

The Set Point Theory is yet another way of looking at the problem. According to this theory, everyone has a biological body weight that is compatible with good health. This weight is maintained by a center in the brain referred to as the "appestat." The appestat "sets" the individual's ideal body weight. When body weight strays too far from the set point, the appestat increases or decreases appetite and burns or conserves the body's store of fat. This theory explains why most of us maintain a fairly stable body weight, despite the day-to-day variation in the type and quantity of food we eat. There seems to be a genetic influence on an individual's biological set point since, as we have seen, there is often a familial tendency toward a heavy or light body build.

If the Set Point Theory is correct, however, why are some people obese? The answer lies in their lifestyle. We are not meant to be sedentary. Primitive people were constantly on the move, either hunting or foraging for food. Lacking this stimulus of physical action, the body senses that something is wrong, the appestat is set to a higher set point, and fat is conserved. The Set Point Theory thus explains why many weight-reduction programs don't work for the truly obese patient. Merely reducing caloric intake will only signal the body to conserve energy and protect its fat stores. If anything, the set point is raised even higher, as a form of protection against the next bout of what the appestat perceives as a period of famine. Only by reprogramming the set point to its normal biological level can weight be permanently reduced. This reprogramming is achieved by a regimen of regular physical exercise combined with a planned diet, the principles of which are a reduction in fat and refined sugars, and an increase in complex carbohydrates such as are found in whole grains, vegetables, and fruit.

Regardless of the obesity theory, the plain fact remains that the only way to maintain a desirable weight is to balance your energy intake and your energy expenditure. A rough guide to the number of calories you should be eating daily is obtained from the following formula: take your desirable weight in kilograms, allow 1 calorie per kilogram per hour over a 24-hour period, and then add 30% to the result. If you are very active, then you may add up to 60%. For example, if your desirable weight is 70 kg, then:

70 kg × 1 × 24		=	1680
+ 30%		=	<u>504</u>
	Total	=	2184

If very active:			
70 kg × 1 × 24		=	1680
+ 60%		=	<u>1008</u>
	Total	=	2688

[Note: Divide your weight in pounds by 2.2 to obtain weight in kilograms.]

Some experts who should know better have dismissed exercise as an essential component of a weight maintenance program. Their argument is that since there are 3,500 calories in a pound (500 grams) of fat, and since a 160-pound (72-kilogram) person burns only 65 calories by walking a mile (1.6 kilometers), then you would have to walk 54 miles (87 kilometers) just to lose one pound (500 grams). This is an oversimplification. Apart from the effect that a regular exercise program may have on lowering your set point, consider a situation in which you reduce your caloric intake by as little as 100 calories per day, and at the same time you walk one mile (1.6 kilometers) daily, to burn 65 calories. In 21 days, you will have lost one pound (500 grams) of body fat. If you walk two miles (three kilometers) a day you will lose one pound (500 grams) of fat in 15 days. Let's say you keep your daily 100-calorie restriction for one year, and walk two miles (three kilometers), five times weekly; at the end of the year you will have lost 20 pounds, or 9 kilograms, of fat. Furthermore, the fat will stay lost. Surely this is the sensible way to lose weight.

Look at it in reverse. It's a popular misconception that obesity is a problem of the middle-aged and elderly. Not so. As a matter of fact, in North America we gain the most weight in our twenties and early thirties. Between the ages of 25 and 35, we put on about 7 to 10 pounds (3 to 5 kilograms). Five percent of that age group gain as much as 30 pounds (14 kilograms). The best way to avoid this is to exercise. Diet alone is not enough. Let us assume that a person becomes only slightly more sedentary over that period, just sufficient for his or her energy intake to exceed the energy expenditure by a mere 100 calories per week. That amounts to 104,000 calories over a 20-year period, which translates into an increase of 30 pounds, or 14 kilograms. So you see, even a relatively mild low-level exercise program can stave off the middle-age bulge. A brisk two- to three-mile (three- to five-kilometer) walk, five times a week, provided it is regular, will burn off excess calories, keep the fat bulge away, and prevent the loss of muscle bulk.

One often hears the plaintive cry, "I eat less than some of my skinny friends, and yet I still get fat." Numerous studies have shown that obese people are past masters at conserving energy. Scientists observing obese children in school and holiday camps have found that they are more sluggish in all physical activities. During field games, they move around as little as possible; during swimming practice, they rest much more frequently than their slim, active friends. As adults, they ride when they could walk, sit when they could stand, and even when sitting move around and fidget less than their thinner colleagues. The bulkier they get, the more difficult and uncomfortable it becomes for them to carry out any form of physical activity, and they are soon caught in a vicious circle. Even though they are eating very little, they are burning even less.

Weight-reduction Strategies

For the truly obese, there are many commercial weight-reduction programs, each claiming to be more successful than the last. North Americans spend about $400 million annually trying to get slim—or about $160 for every pound lost (or $352 for every kilogram)! In general, however, the emphasis is placed entirely on reducing caloric intake. Some programs pay lip service to energy expenditure, offering brief and cursory advice to increase daily physical activities, but rarely is any effort made to draw up an exercise training program tailored to the client's needs. These diets can be categorized broadly into two groups: fad diets and semistarvation diets.

The best-known fad diets advocate a low-carbohydrate, medium- to high-fat, high-protein combination. Initial weight loss may be dramatic, but this is largely due to water loss. The body stores carbohydrate in the muscles and the liver in the form of glycogen. The maximum glycogen storage capacity is 500 grams, or 1 pound. Each gram of glycogen is chemically bound to 3 grams of water, for a total of 1.5 kilograms or 3.5 pounds of water. With a shortage of carbohydrate in the diet, the reserve store of glycogen is quickly called upon, and as it is used it releases its water content to be excreted by the kidneys. Thus, the initial apparently easy loss of weight is not a loss of fat but of water and can be rapidly replaced. Only after the glycogen stores are depleted, and in the absence of a balanced diet, does the body start to use its fat stores. Not only that, but it also breaks down muscle tissue, with resultant muscle wasting, weakness, and severe fatigue. The substances released from the breakdown of fat and muscle tissue can also cause a series of side effects such as acetonelike breath, nausea, headaches, fatigue, and stomach upsets. Even after all this, studies have shown that the weight loss achieved is never permanent.

The semistarvation diets are generally used only in cases of severe obesity, where body fat exceeds 40% to 50% of the total weight. These are usually carried out in a hospital, or under a doctor's supervision. Calories are drastically reduced in an attempt to force the body to burn its excess fat. Again, there is inevitable muscle wasting due to protein breakdown. Supplementing with vitamins and minerals, particularly potassium, is essential. Basic protein needs are satisfied by protein-containing food, or by use of a protein drink. Weight loss can be dramatic, up to 11 pounds (5 kilograms) in the first week, and 5 pounds (2 kilograms) every week thereafter. Constant blood checks are necessary in order to determine mineral loss, and supplemental minerals and vitamins are given accordingly. After about two to three months, the patient is gradually weaned on to a more balanced weight maintenance regimen. Initial results are good, but again, these are rarely long-lasting. Some people have questioned the safety of this approach, especially when it is self-administered. Over the years, a number of deaths have occurred from cardiac complications during the diet.

In the final analysis, a balanced low-calorie diet is the most reasonable approach to weight reduction. The makeup of the diet should be approximately 50% carbohydrate, 30% fat (10% animal and 20% vegetable or fish), and 20% protein. It should typically allow for 1,200 calories a day, with an additional 30% to 60% depending on how active the patient is. The vitamin and mineral content should be adequate, and an accompanying physical training program specifically designed for the obese should always be prescribed. The aim should be to lose no more than 2 pounds (1 kilogram) a week.

Before leaving this topic, two words of caution. Although millions of North Americans are overly fat, there are many others, particularly young women, who strive for what they consider to be the perfect body. Even though they are a desirable weight, they perceive themselves to be fat and succumb to eating disorders such as anorexia nervosa and bulimia. It can only be hoped that a change in our cultural values and a stepped-up health education program will counteract this. Another cause for concern is the possible adverse consequences of losing and then gaining weight as a result of a series of unsuccessful dietary programs. This "yo-yo" effect has been the subject of a number of medical articles in recent years. Although not entirely conclusive, the data strongly suggest that this type of weight fluctuation is associated with an increase in fatal and nonfatal heart attacks.

OTHER POSSIBLE RISK FACTORS

Fibrinogen
In Chapter 2, I described how the formation of a blood clot on top of a coronary atherosclerotic deposit (coronary thrombosis) leads to a heart attack. The clotting mechanism is a complex one, involving the interaction of blood platelets and two protein particles in the blood called thrombin and fibrinogen. Once the platelets clump

together, they start a series of reactions in which thrombin acts on the fibrinogen particles, joining them in long threads of fibrin. The fibrin threads form a meshwork that tangles and traps more platelets and red blood cells to form a firm clot.

A growing number of prospective studies from the United Kingdom, Sweden, and Germany have consistently shown that a high level of fibrinogen in the blood, just like a high blood cholesterol level, is a major independent risk factor not only for a first heart attack but also for a recurrent attack. In fact, it is claimed by some that it is a better predictor than cholesterol. Yet, fibrinogen is still a "new" risk factor, and there is still much we need to learn about it. Is it a truly independent predictor of coronary heart disease or does it operate through some other known risk factor? For instance, smoking is a major cause of high fibrinogen levels, and this could explain to a large extent why it is a risk factor for heart disease. On the other hand, it should be noted that high fibrinogen levels are associated with heart attacks in nonsmokers as well as smokers.

If we accept that there is a causal link between cardiovascular disease and fibrinogen, the next step is to determine how to lower it. There is general agreement that stopping smoking is very effective; ex-smokers' fibrinogen levels are virtually the same as those of persons who have never smoked. Regular exercise has been shown to be associated with a significant decrease in fibrinogen levels. There is also evidence that moderate alcohol consumption lowers fibrinogen in healthy individuals, although this needs to be tested in controlled clinical trials. Some studies suggest that stress increases fibrinogen, although there is no evidence to show that relaxation programs normalize it. Neither does diet have any effect. As for drugs, there is no specific substance taken by mouth that selectively and safely lowers fibrinogen, although two of the fibrate group of drugs (see page 156) fenofibrate and bezafibrate, used to reduce cholesterol levels, have been shown to have some fibrinogen-lowering effect as well. Conversely, the most potent group of cholesterol-lowering drugs, the statins (page 156), are ineffective in this regard.

Of course, further research is required to test whether lowering fibrinogen actually reduces the occurrence of heart disease. If this proves to be so, then we will need to routinely measure fibrinogen levels, just as we measure cholesterol and blood pressure. That will require standardization of methods of measurement, a lengthy process in itself.

Homocysteine

Homocysteine is one of a series of substances produced by the body as it digests and metabolizes protein. In the very rare condition called homocystinuria, the normal chain of events in protein breakdown is interrupted, excessive amounts of homocysteine accumulate in the blood, and large quantities spill over into the urine; hence the name homocystinuria. Sufferers from this genetic defect develop a particularly severe and widespread aggressive form of atherosclerosis, and unless detected and treated early in infancy often die from coronary heart disease or stroke in their early thirties. There is now considerable evidence to show that even mild to moderately elevated homocysteine in otherwise healthy individuals is a strong independent risk factor for cardiovascular disease, and that this is associated with low blood levels of folic acid, and to a lesser extent, vitamin B6 and B12. In 1970 a large Canadian study measured serum folate levels in 5,000 men and women and followed them for 15 years. It found that those with the lowest folate levels had a 69% greater incidence of fatal heart attack compared with those with the highest levels.

In 1997, the *Journal of the American Medical Association*

published the results of a large European study involving nineteen medical centres and nine countries, which showed that subjects with blood homocysteine levels in the top fifth of the population studied had a 120% greater risk of cardiovascular disease than the other four-fifths. The risk associated with elevated homocysteine was higher in women than men. A small number of subjects in the study were taking a vitamin supplement containing folic acid, vitamin B6, and vitamin B12; their risk of cardiovascular events was 62% less than those not taking vitamins. This report, together with others which appeared earlier, is certainly destined to bring homocysteine to the attention of the popular press and the media in general. We still need to determine the precise mechanism by which homocysteine causes atherosclerosis, although experiments have shown that in high concentration it has the capacity to damage the endothelial lining of blood vessels, increase the tendency for the blood to clot, and interact with cholesterol particles in such a way as to facilitate their ability to penetrate the vessel wall. Given that potential, homocysteine could emerge as a risk factor as dangerous as elevated cholesterol levels. In fact, one study found that for every 10% increase in homocysteine levels there is a corresponding 10% rise in the risk of coronary heart disease; another that a 5 micromole per liter increase in blood homocysteine is equivalent to an increase in cholesterol level of 0.5 mmol/L (19 mg/dL).

Why, then, is homocysteine not listed as a major risk factor, with recommendations for population screening and treatment? Because we are living in the age of evidence-based medicine—and just be glad we are. Incontrovertible proof is needed that a risk factor *causes* a disease and is not just associated with it, and that a specific treatment for the risk factor is effective and safe. This requires large well-designed human studies, and until they are completed, advice must be tinged with caution.

Therefore, at this point in time, measurement of homocysteine levels is not part of a routine laboratory assessment. It can be done but is a complicated process. It probably is warranted in special cases, such as someone who has a strong family history of premature heart disease, or a young patient with coronary disease and no apparent classical risk factors. Then there is another problem. As yet there is no clearly defined level which has been proven to be desirable or above which we should start treatment (although there is some evidence that fasting levels above 12 micromoles per liter might constitute a risk). Also, proof is needed that lowering homocysteine levels reduces risk. Finally, assuming that folic acid is effective as a treatment object, how much should we take; daily dosages as low as 400 micrograms and as high as 5 mg have been used in a variety of reported studies.

While we await answers to all these questions, what can we do to protect ourselves? The first step is to ensure that we get enough folate and vitamin B6 in our diet, and both are present in whole grains, wheat bran, brewer's yeast, dark green leafy vegetables, cottage cheese, and beans (in the U.S. folate will be added to flour by 1998). Vitamin B12 is found in large amounts in foods that might be a problem for people with high cholesterol levels. These are liver, kidney, milk, eggs, and cheese. However, poultry, shellfish, fortified cereals and fortified soy products also contain B12. If you feel you are not taking adequate amounts of these foodstuffs, then you might consider a vitamin supplement containing 400 micrograms of folate, as well as the recommended daily allowance of vitamins B6 and B12.

Infections

For years medical scientists have wondered whether coronary artery disease may be due to common chronic bacterial or viral infections, which may act by damaging the endothelial layer and allowing the passage of cholesterol particles into the vessel wall. Until recently, evidence for this theory has been inconclusive, but now there are more convincing reports suggesting an association between coronary atherosclerosis and a bacteria called chlamydia pneumoniae. This organism causes a mild respiratory chest infection, which usually causes only minor symptoms and generally clears up without treatment. Infection leads to the development of antibodies to chlamydia pneumoniae and since about 50% of the population over the age of 50 possess these antibodies, it seems that the infection is quite common. Studies have shown that patients with established coronary artery disease have high levels of antibodies to chlamydia, and that individuals with high readings are twice as likely to develop heart disease as those with low readings. Further support for the chlamydia theory comes from the discovery of the bacteria in the scavenger cells and smooth muscle cells of atherosclerotic plaques obtained from patients with coronary artery disease. Of course, their presence doesn't *prove* that they play any part in the formation of the plaque. Conversely, they may initiate an inflammatory reaction that lays the artery wall open to invasion by cholesterol-laden cells. The chlamydia theory has a number of attractions. The infection is common, as is the incidence of coronary heart disease; high levels of antibodies are a marker for infection and for heart disease; and the bacteria or its antibodies have the potential for inflaming and damaging blood vessel walls. The next step will be to see if aggressive treatment of individuals with antibodies, using anti-chlamydia antibiotics, is associated with a reduction in future cardiovascular events.

We have covered a lot in this chapter, and before closing I think a short summary of the topics discussed is in order.

• We have learned that the epidemic of coronary artery

disease that commenced in the 1920s affects mostly middle-aged men.

- Women in their child-bearing years are relatively immune, but this immunity declines after menopause.
- Medical science has established that those most likely to develop the disease have high blood cholesterol, are cigarette smokers, and often suffer from high blood pressure.
- Diabetes is strongly associated with coronary disease, especially in women.
- Obesity, particularly of the abdominal variety, is another risk factor.
- There seems to be little evidence that there is such a thing as a true coronary-prone personality, but there is a basis for believing that constant stress can ultimately lead to a heart attack.
- Heredity plays a strong role in a small proportion of patients with coronary disease; for the majority, environmental factors far outweigh the genetic aspect.
- Fibrinogen, homocysteine, and bacterial infections are all emerging as possible risk factors, but more research is required before they can be incorporated into a practical strategy for prevention.

It remains for us to discuss in more detail two other very important risk factors, hypercholesterolemia and sedentary lifestyle. Since, as Shakespeare said, "Delays have dangerous ends," let us proceed forthwith to these topics.

4. The Cholesterol Story

If a creature from outer space were to make a tour of our supermarkets and grocery stores, it might conclude that one of our planet's major toxic substances was something called cholesterol. After all, package after package of foodstuffs proudly announce that their contents are "cholesterol-free" or contain "no cholesterol." That same creature, were it to read a medical textbook, would be confused and mystified to learn that cholesterol is not a fat, but a combination of fat and alcohol, and that it is an essential constituent of all the cells of our body, particularly those that make up the tissues of our brain, spinal cord, and nerves. It is also a major ingredient of bile juice and helps to manufacture our body's supply of cortisone and sex hormones. Finally, it forms a protective layer in the skin, preventing the absorption of dangerous acids and solvents into the bloodstream as well as loss of body moisture into the surrounding air.

Without cholesterol, the human body could not survive. Cholesterol is widely distributed in nature and can be found in all animal products, particularly egg yolk and organ meats such as liver, kidney, and brain. We really don't need cholesterol in our diet, since our body can manufacture its own. This process takes place in the liver, which is capable of synthesizing up to six times more cholesterol daily than is found in the average Western diet.

If cholesterol is so vital to our health, how is it that products that have "no cholesterol" are widely advertised as being good for us? I explain this strange paradox to my patients by taking a look at how medical scientists sought to solve the puzzle of atherosclerosis.

Early Studies
As I pointed out previously, scientists first discovered that atherosclerotic deposits contained large quantities of cholesterol. Was is possible, they asked, that animals fed a diet high in cholesterol might develop atherosclerosis? The first answer to that question was published in 1908. It turned out that rabbits could develop severe atherosclerosis if they were given a diet rich in egg yolks, a prolific source of cholesterol. Of course, rabbits are not humans, and it was argued by many that, since they are vegetarians, the addition of any animal or animal product to their diet would be bound to cause some form of abnormality. Nevertheless, by the mid-1930s, as a result of these early experiments, atherosclerosis was thought to be a metabolic disease, caused by a defect in the manner in which the body either made or stored cholesterol. Finding a high level of cholesterol in the blood of people with coronary heart disease would, scientists felt, prove the theory.

For this reason, the principal investigators of the famous Framingham Study decided to include high blood cholesterol levels, together with cigarette smoking and elevated blood pressure, as the possible risk factors they wished to investigate. After all, it was fairly easy to measure blood cholesterol. The simple laboratory procedure involved had been used for years to diagnose various diseases of the liver, kidneys, and thyroid. Why not see if it had any value as a marker for the rapidly increasing disease, coronary atherosclerosis?

If the test had been around for so long, you may ask, why hadn't doctors already noticed that patients with high cholesterol levels were susceptible to subsequent heart attacks? The reason for the oversight lies in the way we determine normal and abnormal laboratory values. Blood cholesterol readings indicative of the noncoronary diseases just mentioned are either very low or very high. Thus, these levels became the reference points for abnormality. As for what is "normal," we also obtained these figures in the usual way—by measuring blood cholesterol in a large number of individuals, of all ages, in our community, and then taking as normal the *average* reading for the different age groups. Unfortunately, there was a potential for error in this method. Assuming that high blood cholesterol is a risk factor for coronary disease, then taking the average reading for a population in which the disease is rampant will give us a figure that might be average, but which certainly will not be "normal" or, to use a more accurate term, *optimal*. For instance, if you look at laboratory manuals printed in the 1970s, you will find that for adults over the age of 30 years, the normal range for blood cholesterol is 6.5 to 7.8 mmol/L (250 to 300 mg/dL).* The early Framingham results, however, showed that middle-aged men with blood cholesterol readings in that range were two to two and a half times more likely to suffer a heart attack in the future. What then was the level below which one was no longer at risk? After more than 30 years of study and observation, this level has recently been established as 5.2 mmol/L (200 mg/dL).

---

*Blood cholesterol levels are now expressed in the new Standard International (SI) units (mmol/L). However, because the older and larger units (mg/dL) are probably more meaningful to the public, they have been retained by the U.S. Public Health authorities for their National Cholesterol Education Program. Both methods of measurement will be quoted throughout this book.

Cholesterol and Diet: the Seven Countries Study

The Framingham Study established that an elevated cholesterol is a strong risk marker for coronary disease. But this knowledge does not tell us how to correct the problem. To do that, we need to understand the link between blood cholesterol and diet. The first study to address this question started in 1958. Known as the Seven Countries Study, it was initiated by the American scientist Dr. Ancel Keys, and its findings are as valid today as they were when they were first published in 1970. Unlike the epidemiological studies referred to earlier in this chapter, which were all within-population, Ancel Keys's study was cross-population, involving approximately 12,000 healthy men between the ages of 40 and 59 from communities in Finland, the Netherlands, Italy, Yugoslavia, Greece, Japan, and the United States. When the study began, subjects were questioned about smoking habits; and their body weight, percent body fat, blood pressure and blood cholesterol were checked, as well as their resting electrocardiograms. They were then followed over a period of ten years for the occurrence of coronary disease. A fairly consistent relationship was found between blood cholesterol and heart disease, not only within the communities themselves, but dramatically so among the different countries. The country with the highest average cholesterol readings, Finland, had the highest incidence of coronary artery disease; in the country with the lowest average cholesterol, Japan, coronary disease was almost unknown. Strong correlations were also found in the United States, the Netherlands, and Italy. These findings confirmed, on an international basis, what had already been discovered in follow-up studies within single communities.

The next major contribution of the Seven Countries Study was that it detected the connection between a country's average cholesterol values and its dietary patterns.

Careful inspection of dietary records and chemical analysis of food samples revealed that the inhabitants of countries where the customary diet was high in fatty foods, such as Finland and the United States, had average blood cholesterols well in excess of 6.5 mmol/L (250 mg/dL) and also suffered excessively from coronary disease. At the other end of the scale were the Japanese subjects who ate little or no fat, had an average blood cholesterol of 4.7 mmol/L (180 mg/dL), and suffered virtually no coronary disease. Of course, as with all multinational studies, there is always the argument that some other cultural factor might be at work, apart from diet. This line of reasoning was directed particularly at the Japanese subjects. However, it was very satisfactorily countered by the Ni-Hon-San Study involving men of Japanese birth who had emigrated to other countries (see page 41).

THE CHEMISTRY OF FATS

Different Types of Fats
The Seven Countries Study identified fat as the major dietary component responsible for increasing blood cholesterol to dangerous levels. However, this information led to further questions: What type of fat? And how much is too much? If we are to understand how Ancel Keys and his co-workers dealt with these problems, we have to take a quick look at the structure and chemistry of fat-containing foods.

The three major components of our daily diet are protein, carbohydrate, and fat. Protein is used for tissue building and repair, carbohydrate for fast muscle action, and fat for prolonged muscle action and long-term energy storage. Pound for pound, fat provides more than twice the energy, or calories, of either of the other two foods. Its very simple chemical structure allows it to fold up easily

for storage purposes. If we eat more protein or carbohydrate than we need, our bodies can convert them into fat,
thus adding even more to our waistlines!

The fat molecule is called a triglyceride and consists of
a combination of glycerol, a substance similar to glycerine,
and three fatty acids (Figure 17). Ordinary everyday fat,
whether it appears on our plate, bulges around our waist,
or is carried around in our blood, is in this form.
Measurement of blood triglyceride levels is a routine procedure, usually carried out at the same time as blood
cholesterol. Hypertriglyceridemia (medical terminology
for high blood triglycerides) is usually associated with
obesity and diabetes. Whether it constitutes an independent risk factor for coronary disease at present remains
uncertain, although recent evidence suggests that this
may well be the case.

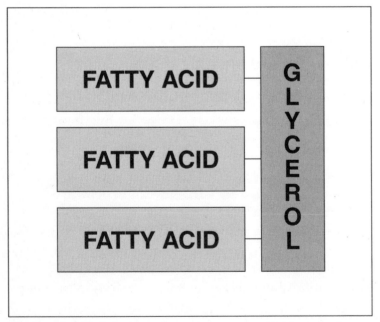

Figure 17: Triglyceride

The active portions of the triglyceride molecule are the fatty acids. As the muscles begin to use up their carbohydrate stores, they rely more and more on fatty acids as their long-term fuel source. As I said, a fatty acid is a very uncomplicated structure, consisting of a series of carbon atoms linked together in a chain, the monotony broken only by the attachment of hydrogen atoms and the occasional oxygen atom. Each carbon atom possesses four hooks, known chemically as bonds, which allow it to attach itself to other atoms. A fatty acid chain in which all the bonds are occupied is referred to as being *saturated*. Empty bonds fold up to form a double bond with their neighbor. Fatty acids with one double bond are referred to as *monounsaturated*, and those with two or more double bonds as *polyunsaturated* (Figure 18).

How does all this chemistry relate to our foodstuffs? Our usual dietary sources of fat are animals, dairy products, grains, and fish. The triglycerides from all these contain varying mixtures of saturated, monounsaturated, and polyunsaturated fatty acids. Animal fats contain a preponderance of saturated fatty acids. Oils from grains, seeds, and fish have a much higher proportion of monounsaturated and polyunsaturated fatty acids. However, there are three exceptions to this, coconut, palm, and palm kernel oils contain large amounts of saturated fatty acids (Figure 19).

Hydrogenation
One further important point. As we all know, the present dietary trend is to substitute vegetable oils for animal fats—that is, to replace saturated with polyunsaturated fatty acids. This trend, however, poses a problem for the food industry. One can use liquid corn oil or safflower oil as a substitute for cooking lard, but what about a liquid substitute for butter? How would you like to *pour* corn oil margarine on your toast in the morning? The solution is

something of a compromise. Food chemists have devised a method of partially saturating the unsaturated vegetable oils. They place the oil in a large tank and bubble hydrogen gas through it. This adds hydrogen atoms to the carbon chain. The process is known as hydrogenation, and the result is a vegetable oil with a higher melting point and a consistency closer to that of an animal fat. It is also easier to package and more appealing to use.

Hydrogenation is also used for another purpose. The empty spaces in the unsaturated fatty acid chain are just a little bit too available to any passing molecule that happens to be homeless at the time. The most commonly available molecule is oxygen; so, over a period of time, the inclusion of oxygen in the carbon chain causes the fatty acid to change its properties. It develops a rather unpleasant odor and taste. In other words, it becomes rancid. Obviously, if you attach hydrogen atoms to the spaces along the chain, you reduce the likelihood of rancidity. In short, if you want to prolong the shelf life of any foodstuff containing an unsaturated fat, you merely hydrogenate that fat.

Hydrogenation, then, certainly has its uses. However, we must never forget that it is a process which converts a polyunsaturated fatty acid into a saturated fatty acid, and that this has to be taken into account when planning a heart-healthy diet.

Dangerous Fats and Safe Fats
Now that we have defined our chemical terms, we can return to the work of Ancel Keys and his colleagues. The Seven Countries Study identified a fatty diet as an apparent cause of high blood cholesterol. This information, however, was not precise enough to be of practical value. Were all fats dangerous, or only certain types of fats? To answer this question, a series of feeding experiments was carried out. Volunteers agreed to follow a number of

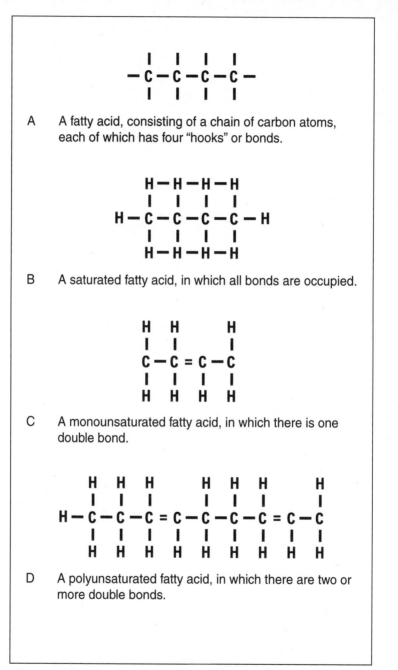

A   A fatty acid, consisting of a chain of carbon atoms, each of which has four "hooks" or bonds.

B   A saturated fatty acid, in which all bonds are occupied.

C   A monounsaturated fatty acid, in which there is one double bond.

D   A polyunsaturated fatty acid, in which there are two or more double bonds.

Figure 18: Fatty Acids

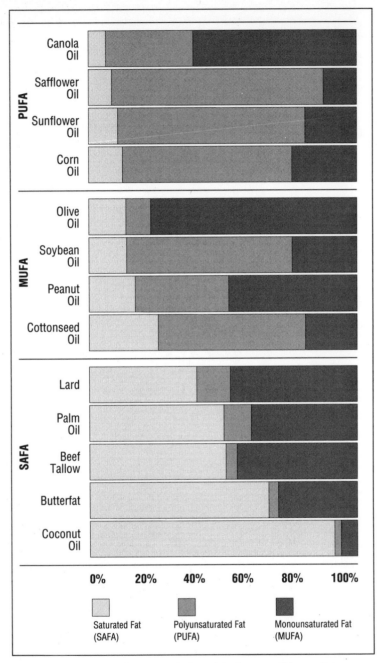

Figure 19: The Types of Fatty Acids Found in Common Dietary Fats

carefully prepared diets in the controlled environment of an institution. Differing quantities and types of fats were included, and blood cholesterol levels were measured regularly. In summary, the following very important findings emerged:

1. Saturated fatty acids, found largely in animal meats and dairy products, raise blood cholesterol.
2. Polyunsaturated fatty acids, found largely in vegetable and fish oils, tend to lower blood cholesterol.
3. Hydrogenated polyunsaturated fatty acids, found in processed foods such as margarine, pastries, cakes, some breakfast cereals, chocolate bars, etc., are artificially saturated, and raise cholesterol to the same extent as natural animal products.
4. Monounsaturated fatty acids, found most commonly in olive oil, are neutral, neither raising nor lowering cholesterol levels.
5. Cholesterol itself, found in all animal meats but in abundance in egg yolk and organ meats such as liver, brain, kidney, and heart, also tends to raise cholesterol in the blood, but not to the same extent as saturated fatty acids.

Good and Bad Cholesterol, and Atherosclerosis
We have seen that cholesterol is an essential component of all animal tissue, particularly that of essential organs such as the brain, skin, and the glands which produce our sex hormones. It acts like a sort of cement, or mortar, strengthening and fortifying the walls of the cells. Cholesterol is a waxy substance, and as such does not dissolve in water. Yet it needs to pass from the liver where it is made or from the gut from which it is absorbed, to and from the various tissues. The body's transport system is the bloodstream, but since blood is 60% water, fats will not dissolve in blood. The problem of how to transport these fats is

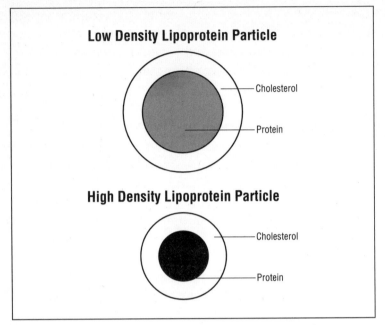

Figure 20: The "Good" (HDL) and the "Bad" (LDL) Lipoprotein

solved by protein particles, called lipoproteins, which act as carriers of cholesterol and triglycerides. By making cholesterol soluble in water, the lipoproteins allow it to be transported through the bloodstream. Although very small, lipoproteins can be subdivided by their size and density into very low density (VLDL), low density (LDL), and high density (HDL) lipoproteins. An analogy for their size and weight might be, respectively, a soccer ball, a baseball, and a billiard ball. Triglycerides are carried almost exclusively by the "soccer ball" or VLDL particles. Cholesterol, on the other hand, can be carried by both the "baseball" LDL and the "billiard ball" HDL particles (Figure 20).

How does this relate to our story? In the early 1980s, the Framingham data clearly demonstrated that those who were at most risk for heart disease were those with high levels of LDL-cholesterol (LDL-C). It is still debated whether LDL-C rather than total cholesterol should be used as the first screening measurement to predict heart disease in the community. LDL-C is a better predictor, but currently it is only measured directly in a research laboratory; in routine clinical practice it is estimated from a formula which takes into account total cholesterol, HDL-C, and triglyceride measurements.

In 1985, Dr. Michael Brown and Dr. Joseph Goldstein were awarded a Nobel Prize for their discovery of LDL-C receptors. You can think of these as sockets situated on the cell wall into which plug the LDL-C particles. The number of receptors are determined genetically, with one gene from each parent. When both genes are defective (homozygous hypercholesterolemia), there is a drastic reduction in the number of LDL-receptors. This genetic defect occurs in about one in a million of the population. In these individuals, cholesterol levels range as high as 25.9 mmol/L (1,000 mg/dL), and fatal heart attacks generally occur in the teens. Where only one gene is defective (heterozygous hypercholesterolemia), a condition occurring in about 1 in 500 people, cholesterol levels exceed 7.8 mmol/L (300 mg/dL), and heart attacks usually occur when they are in their thirties or forties. In either form, even when blood cholesterol levels are optimal, there are insufficient receptors to accept a normal complement of LDL-C particles. As a result, the spare LDL-C particles circulate in the blood, becoming increasingly numerous and ready to contribute to the formation of an atheroma.

This discovery had implications not only for hypercholesterolemia, but also for the population as a whole, since it enabled us to see the problem of high blood cholesterol in terms of an imbalance between particles and receptors. Let us say that you possess a normal complement of LDL-C receptors, but eat a diet high in animal fat. For some reason that we have not as yet discovered, our liver then commences to make excess cholesterol. This excess is then attached to LDL particles, which appear in large quantities in the blood. A proportion of these would soon occupy all the available receptors, leaving the remainder to be carried around aimlessly in the blood, unable to find a parking space.

In this eventuality, one of the body's defense mechanisms takes over. The excess LDL-C particles are picked up by a form of white blood cell called a *scavenger cell*, which takes them out of the bloodstream and deposits them into special *scavenger receptors* which are located in the blood vessel wall just under the endothelial lining. Areas where the endothelial lining is already damaged by, for example, some toxic agents such as cigarette smoke, or the effects of high blood pressure, are often easiest for the scavenger cells to traverse. Unlike the Brown and Goldstein LDL-C receptors, which accept just so much LDL-C and no more, the scavenger receptors have no such mechanism. They will continue to gorge on LDL-C-laden scavenger cells as long as there is excess cholesterol to scavenge until, like an overstretched balloon, they burst, releasing liquid fat into the surrounding tissue of the vessel wall.

This is the start of a chain of events that leads to the atherosclerotic plaque. The body forms a fibrous cap over the bulging fat mass in an attempt to ward it off from the lumen of the blood vessel, and prevent it from leaking into the bloodstream. From time to time, this is only partially successful, and when small amounts of fat ooze through a crack in the cap and mix with the blood, a clot forms. Given time this becomes solid (another of the body's defenses), but the net result is an increase in the size of the plaque, which may eventually completely obstruct the blood flow. This explains the clinical picture of increasing anginal symptoms over a period of years, followed by a heart attack.

Another scenario is one that can occur when the plaque

is fresh, and the fibrous cap is in the early stages of for-mation. It is then barely capable of retaining the bulging fat mass within its walls. If it now ruptures, the ensuing clot may be so large that it instantly and completely blocks the blood flow and causes a sudden heart attack, often in an individual who has previously been apparently quite healthy. In fact, the only previous abnormal physical find-ing may be an elevated blood cholesterol! The disturbing fact is that at this dangerous stage of its early formation the plaque is often so small that it may not even show on a coronary angiogram. As we have seen, the way to avoid all of this is to ensure that our diet does not contain too much saturated fat. This will ensure that our total choles-terol does not rise too high.

From the Framingham data we have an optimal figure of 5.2 mmol/L (200 mg/dL) or less for *total cholesterol*. We know that approximately 50%–60% of this cholesterol is normally transported in the blood by LDL particles. Thus, a quick calculation gives us an optimal value for LDL-C of 2.6–3.2 mmol/L (100–120 mg/dL).

What about the smaller, heavier HDL-C particles? What role do they play? In the mid-1970s, evidence began to accumulate suggesting that HDL particles are respon-sible for picking up any unwanted additional LDL-C before it is engulfed by scavenger cells, and transporting it back to the liver in the form of HDL-C, where it com-bines with the bile juice and is excreted in the bowel. This would imply that people with high levels of HDL-C could dispose of excess LDL-C particles and would therefore be less likely to develop coronary artery disease. This theory has been supported by epidemiological evidence, show-ing that there is an inverse relationship between HDL-C level and coronary disease; that is, the higher the HDL-C, the less the risk of a heart attack. Males before puberty and females before menopause have high HDL-C, after which the level drops and they both become susceptible to heart disease. Diabetics, cigarette smokers, and the obese also have low HDL-C. Whereas dietary measures can raise or lower LDL-C, HDL-C does not seem to be affected by these measures. It seems to respond favorably only to a regular exercise program and certain drugs. The optimal value for HDL-C is 0.9 mmol/L (35 mg/dL) or greater, although for premenopausal women I feel the figure should be closer to 1.4 mmol/L (54 mg/dL).

I personally believe, at least in terms of blood cholesterol measurements, that the best predictor of a future heart attack is the ratio of total cholesterol to HDL-C. This ratio is calculated by dividing total cholesterol by HDL-C; for example, total cholesterol 6.1 (240) ÷ HDL-C 1.6 (60) = 4:1. A ratio of 5 for men and 4.5 for women represents average risk. The total cholesterol/HDL-C ratio should be as close to 3.5 as possible. It should be noted that while total cholesterol and HDL-C are very reliable measurements in the hands of any general medical laboratory, LDL-C is not and has to be calculated from a formula that takes into account TC, HDL-C, and triglycerides. The suggested strategy for using these measurements to lower blood cholesterol in the population at large has been initiated by the United States National Cholesterol Education Program and, to a varying degree, has been adopted by most countries, including Canada and the United Kingdom. An outline of this approach will be presented later in the chapter.

Let's pause for a moment and marshal the facts we have established so far. Starting with the early laboratory observations that atherosclerosis could be artificially induced in animals by feeding them a diet high in cholesterol and fat, we progressed to the studies, such as the Framingham Study, that noted a relationship between high blood cholesterol and the incidence of coronary artery disease. Ancel Keys, through the Seven Countries Study, demonstrated the link between blood cholesterol, dietary fat intake, and death from coronary heart disease. Feeding experiments then identified dietary saturated (animal) fat as the culprit, with polyunsaturated (vegetable and fish) oils exerting a partial protective effect. Finally, we have established optimal levels for the various cholesterol measurements. Now it remains to look at the dietary strategy that will allow us to attain and maintain those levels.

Essentials of a Healthy Heart Diet

There are some who advocate complete elimination of animal fat from the diet, and for those of us who can follow a rigid vegetarian diet this may have considerable health benefits. Indeed, it may be an essential part of an overall strategy for those with a bad personal or family history of coronary heart disease. It seems to me, however, that for most individuals the American Heart Association (AHA) Step I or Step II diet (see Appendix H), together with cholesterol-lowering medication if indicated, is a more prudent and realistic option. The attraction of the AHA diet is that it is so easy to follow, particularly now that food labelling is becoming more meaningful in terms of fat content. The aim is to define the optimal daily intake of saturated fat. This will depend, of course, on the total daily caloric intake, which in turn will depend on the energy requirements of the individual. For example, whereas someone engaged in heavy manual labor might need to eat as much as 4,000 calories daily, the average middle-aged sedentary worker will only require about 2,000 calories. The AHA Step I diet recommends that only 10% of the total caloric intake come from saturated fat; the Step II that the maximum permitted daily intake of saturated fat be only 7%. Thus for a 2,000 calorie daily intake, a Step I diet will allow 10% of 2,000, or 200 calories and for a Step II diet, 7% of 2,000, or 140 calories.

Now, although physiologists and food scientists think

in terms of calories when they calculate energy expenditure and food intake, the rest of us think in terms of more meaningful amounts, such as grams. How do we convert 200 calories, or 140 calories, to grams? Quite simply. There are 9.5 calories in 1 gram of fat. Thus, 200 calories of fat equals approximately 20 grams, and 140 calories approximately 15 grams. Just remember that, assuming you are middle-aged and sedentary, you should not eat more than 20 grams of saturated fat (or if you have been told by your doctor to follow a Step II diet, 15 grams of saturated fat), daily.

Calculating Your Fat Budget			
		%Fat	
Daily Intake	**10%**	**20%**	**30%**
Calories	Grams of Fat (%total calories ÷ 9.0)		
1800	20	40	60
2000	22	44	67
2200	24	49	73
2400	26	53	80

(Table 2)

This is where the ability to read a label comes in. The label should state the number of grams of polyunsaturated, monounsaturated, and saturated fat in a serving, and it should also specify the size of a serving, e.g., tablespoons, ounces, etc. Whether or not it gives the proportion of hydrogenated fat or natural fat hardly matters. The origin of the saturated fat is not as important as the total amount in a serving. American labeling laws are excellent in this regard. At the moment, Canadian law has some catching up to do, but hopefully we will hasten to follow the American example. It makes things so much easier. You buy a package of high-fat cheese and you discover from the label that a 1-ounce serving contains 6 grams of saturated fat; eat 3 ounces and you have almost reached your total saturated fat allowance for the day. On the other hand, a low-fat cheese may only contain half a gram of saturated fat per ounce; eat 3 ounces and you still have about 18 grams of your daily ration of saturated fat left. What about non-packaged foodstuffs such as a cut of beef or pork, bacon, ham, etc.? Fortunately, there is a multitude of low-cost cookbooks on the market which will give you the saturated fat content of a serving of almost every kind of food you can imagine.

HOW DO WE LOWER BLOOD CHOLESTEROL?

If Ancel Keys's observation is correct, that a diet high in animal fat can cause hypercholesterolemia and eventually lead to coronary atherosclerosis, then by the same token lowering blood cholesterol to optimal levels should reduce the incidence of coronary disease. This has been put to the test by a series of prospective clinical trials. They fall into one of two categories, depending on whether the cholesterol-lowering was attempted by altering the diet, or by giving a drug.

Dietary Intervention
Three early studies, the Finnish Mental Hospital Study, the Los Angeles Veteran Study, and the Oslo Primary Prevention Trial, involving some 4,000 healthy men, showed that a diet low in animal fat resulted in a reduction in blood cholesterol levels, and that this was associated with a significant drop in the incidence of fatal and nonfatal heart attacks. A British study, the Diet and Reinfarction Trial (DART), which involved 2,000 men who had already suffered a heart attack, showed that those who had a meal containing a serving of oily fish two to three times a week had a 29% reduction in death from all

causes over a two-year follow-up period. But perhaps the most impressive results come from the Lyon Diet Heart Study which investigated the effects of a Mediterranean-type diet (more vegetables, fruit, fish, canola and olive oils, canola-oil margarine, and less meat) on a group of 300 heart attack survivors. Compared with an age-matched group of 300 controls, those on the diet had 70% fewer nonfatal heart attacks and 80% fewer cardiovascular deaths over the follow-up period of five years.

Thus there seems little doubt that adherence to a diet low in saturated fat can reduce cholesterol levels and the risk of coronary heart disease. However, dietary trials have been relatively few in number for the following reasons. They cannot be "blinded," i.e., each subject knows whether or not he or she is on the experimental diet and therefore the "placebo effect" cannot be avoided. Furthermore, adherence to the diet is very difficult to monitor; one has only the subject's word as to adherence. Finally, large-scale trials require large investments of money, and since food cannot be patented, the only source of money is government or some philanthropic group. Which brings us to the drug trials.

Drug Trials
The use of drugs to test the cholesterol theory has obvious advantages. It is easier to take a medication than to change one's diet, and therefore there is less of a problem with compliance. A placebo can be used for the control group, and the trial can be "blinded"; the patients do not know which group they are in, and neither do their doctors. This eliminates the possible influence of suggestion.

From a historical viewpoint, the two most important drug trials of the 1980s were the American Lipid Research Clinic's Coronary Drug Prevention Trial, referred to simply as the LRC Trial, and the Finnish Helsinki Trial. The LRC Trial involved approximately 4,000 healthy men who had high blood cholesterol levels. They were divided into two groups, half receiving a cholesterol-lowering drug called cholestyramine (Questran), and the other a placebo; the entire group was followed from 1973 to 1983. There was no significant difference between the two groups in fatal and nonfatal heart attacks if looked at separately. However, if we add fatal and nonfatal together, then there is a statistically significant difference between the two groups, in favor of those receiving cholestyramine.

The Helsinki Trial also involved 4,000 men with high blood cholesterol levels, and the drug used was gemfibrozil (Lopid). As in the LRC Study, there was no difference between the groups with regard to fatal or nonfatal heart attacks alone, but there was a significant difference in favor of the treated group when the two were added together. Thus the message from the 1980s trials was encouraging, but for some advocates of the cholesterol theory, not as conclusive as they might have wished.

The 1990s changed all that, with the use of the newer potent cholesterol-lowering "statin" drugs (see Chapter 6). The first of these was lovastatin (Mevacor), soon to be followed by simvastatin (Zocor), and pravastatin (Pravachol). These drugs are known technically as HMG-CoA reductase inhibitors, and they act by preventing the liver from making excessive amounts of LDL-C; they also bring about a modest rise in HDL-C. Despite initial fears, experience to date suggests that they have few or no harmful side effects. Their effectiveness was first demonstrated in a large-scale European trial, the Scandinavian Simvastatin Survival Study (referred to as the 4S), the results of which were published in 1994 in the prestigious medical journal, *The Lancet*. Patients with angina or a previous heart attack and high cholesterol levels (6.7 mmol/L, 260 mg/dL) treated with simvastatin (Zocor), achieved a substantial reduction in total cholesterol and LDL-C. This was associated with highly significant reductions in fatal and nonfatal heart attacks, strokes, and the need for bypass surgery (Table 3). A similar study, the Cholesterol and Recurrent Events Trial (CARE) was published shortly thereafter. It also involved patients with established coronary artery disease, but with normal cholesterol levels (5.4 mmol/L, 209 mg/dL) and treated them with pravastatin (Pravachol). The results were just as impressive as those of the 4S, with the added discovery that the effect of the cholesterol-lowering treatment on the occurrence of coronary events was greater among women than among men (a 46% reduction in coronary events compared with 20%) (Table 4). Any doubts with regard to the benefit of cholesterol-lowering in patients with coronary disease have now been thoroughly dispelled by the results of both of these trials.

What about the effect of cholesterol-lowering on *healthy* subjects whose cholesterol levels are considered high, i.e., the problem which the LRC Trial had previously attempted to answer, with only qualified success. After all, screening the population for those at high risk for a heart attack because of elevated cholesterol is only justified if there is a proven treatment which can reduce that risk. A major step in this direction was provided by the West of Scotland Coronary Prevention Study (WOSCOPS), which demonstrated that healthy hypercholesterolemic men treated with pravastatin achieved reductions in total cholesterol and LDL-C similar to those produced in 4S and CARE, with an associated 31% reduction in risk of nonfatal or fatal heart attacks. The need for coronary artery bypass graft surgery and the incidence of total mortality from all causes was also reduced (Table 5).

Although the 4S, CARE and WOSCOPS studies are officially ended, published follow-ups of the subjects continue to show increased survival and fewer coronary events in the treated groups. It would be impossible to overestimate the implications of these reports on the practice of cardiology today. We now have solid scientific evidence that lowering total cholesterol and LDL-C will substantially reduce the incidence of heart disease. I say substantially—not entirely. There are still the other risk factors to be taken into account when designing a treatment strategy, as we shall now see.

Variable	Treated vs Usual Care %
LDL-cholesterol	-35
Fatal heart attack	-32
CABG surgery	-37
Stroke	-30
All coronary events	-33 Men; -35 Women
< 60 years	-38
>60 years	-28
	(Lancet, 1994)

Table 3: The Scandinavian Simvastation Survival Study (4S)

Variable	Treated vs Usual Care %
Total cholesterol	-20
LDL-cholesterol	-32
Fatal heart attack	-20
CABG surgery	-26
Angioplasty	-23
Stroke	-31
All coronary events	-20 (Men)
	-46 (Women)
	(NEJM, 1996)

Table 4: Cholesterol and Recurrent Events Trial (CARE)

Variable	Treated vs Usual Care %
Total cholesterol	-20
LDL cholesterol	-26
Fatal heart attacks	-28
Fatal + nonfatal heart attacks	-31
CABG surgery	-37
	(NEJM, 1995)

Table 5: West of Scotland Coronary Prevention Study (WOSCOPS)

Attain ideal body weight: diet & exercise

Reduce: total fat calories to less than 30% of total intake

Reduce: saturated (mainly animal) to less than 10% of total intake, substitute monounsat. and polyunsat. fats (vegetable, olive & fish oils)

Reduce: dietary choresterol to less than 300 mg/day

Increase: complex carbohydrates & fibers (fruit, cereals, vegetables)

Table 6: Lipid-lowering Diet: General Advice

Dealing with Detection and Treatment of High Blood Cholesterol

The American National Cholesterol Education Program (NCEP) was first published in 1988, with a later report in 1994. With minor modifications, it has been adopted in practically all countries where coronary heart disease is a problem, which means most of the industrialized world. It provides physicians with a practical plan for detecting and treating those at risk of developing heart disease because of elevated blood cholesterol. The first step in the screening process is to determine the levels of total cholesterol and HDL cholesterol from a blood sample taken from the vein in front of the elbow and then analyzed in the laboratory. Alternatively, a portable cholesterol analyzer now on the market gives a reading from a finger-prick sample within two minutes, and in our experience at the Toronto Centre, can be almost as accurate as the laboratory reading. These measurements, incidentally, can be made in the non-fasting state. Screening, of course, is only a means to an end. The next step is to determine the cholesterol level, or cut-off point, above which strategies to reduce cholesterol are prescribed. The NCEP has identified a total blood cholesterol of 5.2 mmol/L (200 mg/dL) or less, and an HDL cholesterol of 0.9 mmol/L (35 mg/dL) or greater, as being desirable, or low risk. Total cholesterol levels between 5.2 mmol/L (200 mg/dL) and 6.2 mmol/L (239 mg/dL) are classified as borderline risk, and those above 6.2 mmol/L (239 mg/dL) as high risk. Those individuals who fall into the low-risk category will require no further action, apart from a repeat cholesterol reading in, say, five years' time. Those at high risk will be entered into a dietary, and if necessary, a drug program.

How do we deal with the borderline group, those between 5.2 mmol/L (200 mg/dL) and 6.2 mmol/L (239 mg/dL)? This is where we have to distinguish between *relative risk* and *attributable risk*. Relative risk is the likelihood of someone with a risk factor, as opposed to someone without that risk factor, developing coronary artery disease. The relative risk of a blood cholesterol concentration of 7.8 mmol/L (300 mg/dL), compared with one of 4.6 mmol/L (178 mg/dL) is about 5:1, or five times higher. However, since only 10% or less of the population have such a markedly elevated blood cholesterol reading, it does not contribute greatly to the overall incidence of the disease. Attributable risk, on the other hand, addresses this issue, and asks the question, at what cholesterol level do most heart attacks occur? According to Dr. William Castelli of the Framingham Study, that figure is 5.8

mmol/L (225 mg/dL), which is almost exactly midway in the NCEP "borderline" risk zone of 5.2 mmol/L (200 mg/dL) to 6.2 mmol/L (239 mg /dL). In fact, more than 50% of fatal heart attacks occur in individuals whose blood cholesterol falls in the borderline range. It may be borderline in terms of relative risk, but its attributable risk is very high. Why is that? Because 25% of the adult population of North America have cholesterol readings in the borderline range, and this group comprises many millions. On the other hand, although over half of fatal heart attack victims will be found to have a borderline cholesterol level, not all of the millions with a borderline reading will necessarily develop coronary artery disease. How do we screen out those who will from those who won't?

This is where we introduce other risk factors into the equation. Individuals with borderline readings should undergo a second screening, this time after fasting overnight. On this occasion LDL cholesterol and triglyceride measurements should be included. Our major focus is now on the LDL-C. A level of 3.4 mmol/L (130 mg/dL) or less is considered desirable, and need not be repeated for five years. Levels between 3.4 mmol/L (130 mg/dL) and 4.1 mmol/L (159 mg/dL) are borderline, and if fewer than two other risk factors are present, then the individual is given advice on a dietary regimen and a physical activity program, and retested in one year. If, however, two or more risk factors are present, or the LDL-C level is greater than 4.1 mmol/L (160 mg/dL), then we are dealing with a high-risk situation; intensive dietary therapy and/or cholesterol-lowering drugs are indicated, the goal being to reduce LDL-C levels to 2.6 mmol/L (100 mg/dL) or less.

All men and women who have proven coronary heart disease should have the full screening, with the goal of reducing their LDL-C to 2.6 mmol/L (100 mg/dL) and increasing their HDL-C to 0.9 mmol/L (35 mg/dL) or greater.

Whereas a diet low in saturated fat will reduce L it will not raise HDL-C. Apart from some medicatio only lifestyle changes that will achieve that desirabɩe eɩɩɑ are quitting smoking, weight reduction if you are obese, and if you are sedentary, starting an exercise program. The second NCEP report, while still pointing out the danger of elevated LDL-C levels, gave considerably more emphasis to HDL-C than the first. In fact, an HDL-C level of 1.6 mmol/L (60 mg/dL) or greater has been designated a "negative" risk factor (See Appendix X).

I believe that future guidelines will accentuate HDL-C readings even further, a viewpoint supported by the Framingham data. For instance, since the last edition of this book in 1992, scientists have identified a smaller, denser LDL-C particle, which is particularly dangerous for the development of atherosclerosis. However, identification of these LDL-C particles by routine laboratory testing is not likely to be available to your doctor for a number of years yet. In the meantime, there is no need for worry. The presence of these small, dense LDL-C particles can be detected by the fact that they are always associated with low levels of HDL-C; measures to reduce total cholesterol (diet and drugs) and to increase HDL-C (exercise, weight loss, stopping smoking, and taking appropriate medications) will be equally effective. A similar situation arises in connection with triglycerides. The NCEP recommends a level of 2.2 mmol/L (200 mg/dL) or less. However, we know that triglyceride particles can occur in two forms, a large, fluffy type, which is harmless and is often increased in vegetarians, and a smaller, more dangerous type, which is a risk factor for heart disease. Again, there is no readily available clinical laboratory test which will distinguish between the two. However, if the triglyceride is greater than 2.2 mmol/L (200 mg/dL) and is associated with an HDL-C less than 0.9 mmol/L (35 mg/dL), then we are dealing with the riskier triglycerides. On the other hand, a strict vegetarian with a triglyceride level of 3.3 mmol/L (300 mg/dL) and an HDL-C level of 1.7 mmol/L (64 mg/dL) need have no fear. In short, the HDL-C reading is very important, and I would advocate that it be a routine measurement, part of the overall cholesterol assessment. I believe that the total-cholesterol/HDL-C ratio is more important than the total-cholesterol reading, particularly in women, and should be taken into account when determining which individuals with a borderline total-cholesterol reading are at high risk.

As for intervention, the NCEP advocates the AHA Step-I or II diet, together with exercise, weight loss, and if necessary, drugs. Table 6 outlines the general lifestyle treatment strategy.

Multiple Risk Factors
The NCEP strategy, while concentrating on cholesterol levels, illustrates the powerful cumulative effect of additional risk factors (Figure 21). What may be less obvious is the multiplicative effect of the presence of a number of risk factors that are only mildly elevated. For instance, you might not think that an individual with a mildly elevated blood cholesterol of 6.2 mmol/L (239 mg/dL) and a borderline-high blood pressure of 150/90 mm Hg, who smokes only five cigarettes a day, would be at high risk for a heart attack, but in fact, when you take all these "mildly" elevated risk factors together, you have a profile of someone with a risk as grave as if they had a blood cholesterol of 7.8 mmol/L (300 mg/dL) or a blood pressure of 180/110 mm Hg, or smoked two packs of cigarettes a day! (Figure 22.)

Multiple Risk Factor Intervention

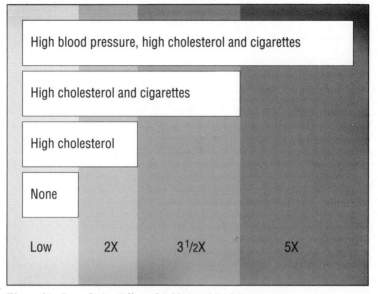

Figure 21: Cumulative Effect of Additional Risk Factors
The individual who exhibits multiple risk factors greatly increases the chance of developing coronary disease.

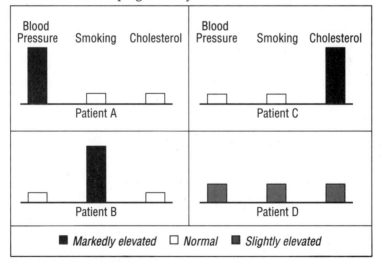

Figure 22: Balancing Risk Factors
Four patients, A, B, C and D have the same risk of developing coronary disease. In the case of patients A, B and C, the presence of one markedly elevated risk factor is obvious. Patient D, with three mildly elevated factors, may not recognize the extent of the risk.

5. Other Dietary Considerations

There have been a number of additions to the original findings of Ancel Keys. None of these, mark you, overshadows the main thrust of his argument: that the single most important dietary cause of hypercholesterolemia is an excess of dietary fat.

Antioxidants
Oxygen is the fuel that sparks all of the body's metabolic processes. However, like all fuels, it can produce undesirable by-products. These are known as oxygen free radicals. They are unstable molecules which are missing one electron. Their harm lies in their ability to interact with other essential molecules in the fat, protein, or DNA of the cell, and steal one of their electrons. The process of oxidation has been likened to rusting, and it is an inevitable feature of life. Humans suffer about 10,000 attacks by oxygen free radicals to their DNA daily. Fortunately, the body can repair the damage by using its inbuilt antioxidant enzymes. However, if these begin to fail or are overwhelmed, oxidation begins to take over, contributing to aging, cancer, and coronary artery disease. Additional

contributors to oxidative stress include smoking, chronic infections, alcohol, environmental pollution, excessive exposure to ultraviolet light, and even bouts of vigorous exhaustive exercise.

Antioxidants work by donating an electron to the oxygen-free radical molecule before it can steal one from a healthy molecule. In a sense they are like mobile SWAT teams, cruising through the tissues of the body looking for oxygen free radicals, and neutralizing them before they can do any damage. In addition to those occurring naturally in the body, dietary antioxidants play a major role in the protective mechanism. Fruits and vegetables contain the largest amounts of these key nutrients, and evidence from nearly 200 studies suggests that inadequate consumption of these foods is consistently linked to higher rates of cancer. While there seems little doubt that these foodstuffs contain antioxidants as yet unknown, those currently attracting attention are vitamin E, vitamin C, beta-carotene, the flavonoids and co-enzyme Q10.

Oxidation plays a major role in the development of coronary atherosclerosis. In fact, it has helped to explain a previously puzzling question about how the LDL-C particles are able to burrow into the coronary artery wall. You will recall how in Chapter 4 we learned that excess LDL-C in the blood was picked up by scavenger cells and deposited in scavenger receptors beneath the endothelial layer of the vessel. The problem is that normal LDL-C is not recognized by the scavengers, and so cannot be picked up and transported across the endothelium. However, if the LDL-C becomes oxidized, then it is readily recognized and engulfed by the scavengers. The susceptibility to oxidation of LDL-C depends on (1) the amount of LDL-C in the blood (an excess, from eating too much animal fat, favouring oxidation), (2) the size of the LDL-C particle (the smaller, denser are more prone to oxidation) and (3) the availability of antioxidants in the tissues. Therefore, antioxidant nutrients that protect tissues against attack by free oxygen radicals are important therapeutically. There is a debate, however, as to whether we should attempt to be getting all our antioxidants in a balanced diet, or whether we should be getting them in the form of supplements. Traditionally, food scientists have always argued in favour of the former, but recent evidence suggests that for many of us, the dietary intake is inadequate. British and European studies have shown that in areas where the incidence of coronary heart disease is high, tissue concentrations of antioxidants are significantly lower than in countries where the incidence of coronary heart disease is low and the consumption of cereals, vegetables and fruits is high, e.g., the Mediterranean countries. An American study found that only 10% of the population were regularly eating the recommended amount of fruit and vegetables. So, while we should be striving to eat a balanced diet, many of us will have to consider supplementation with the major antioxidant vitamins.

Vitamin E, first discovered in the 1920s at the University of California at Berkeley and championed for many years by Dr. Evan Shute of London, Ontario, as a potent antioxidant, finally seems to have come into its own. The scientific basis for its benefit in coronary heart disease lies in the fact that it is a fat-soluble vitamin, and as such is incorporated directly into the LDL-C particle. Once there it can immediately provide the missing electrons for the oxygen free radicals, rendering them harmless, and so blocking the formation of the dangerous oxidized LDL-C. Vitamin E also reduces the blood's ability to clot, which may be another factor in preventing heart attacks.

In 1993, the results of two large American studies, the Nurses' Health Study and the Health Professionals' Follow-up Study, were published in the *New England Journal of Medicine*. The former enrolled 87,000 healthy women, followed them for eight years, and found that women taking 100 international units (I.U.) of vitamin E or more in supplement form for at least two years had a 40% lower risk of developing coronary heart disease, in contrast with those not taking the supplement. One might assume that this is overwhelming evidence in favour of everyone taking vitamin E, but not necessarily so. Only 15% of the nurses were actively taking the vitamin, and of these, there were fewer smokers, more who exercised regularly, and more taking hormone replacement therapy. This suggests that the vitamin takers were more health-conscious, and therefore more healthy to start with, and so not necessarily representative of the whole population.

The Health Professionals' Follow-up Study evaluated the effect of dietary supplements on 40,000 healthy men over a period of 10 years. Once again, those taking 100 I.U. or more of vitamin E in supplement form had a 40% lower risk of developing coronary heart disease, and the protective effect persisted even in the presence of other major risk factors such as smoking and hypercholesterolemia. Interestingly, men who relied entirely on dietary sources of vitamin E did not obtain a protective effect, reinforcing a very strong argument in favour of supplementation. It should also be noted that in both studies supplementation with small amounts of vitamin E, less than 100 I.U., was ineffectual; which probably explains the failure of a randomized controlled Finnish trial which used low-dose preparations of vitamin E to show any effect on the incidence of heart attacks. A 1996 report described the effect of vitamin E supplementation on 11,000 elderly persons aged 67 to 105 years, followed for eight years. Again, there was a 40% reduction in deaths from coronary disease compared with those not taking the supplement.

What about the use of vitamin E in individuals who have already developed coronary heart disease? This was the object of a British study, the Cambridge Heart

Antioxidant Study (CHAOS), published in *The Lancet* in 1996. Two thousand patients were enrolled, half randomized to 400 to 800 I.U. of vitamin E daily, and the other half to a placebo. Over a one-year period, the effect of vitamin E was to reduce the incidence of nonfatal, but not fatal, heart attack by 77%. The failure to achieve a reduction in the incidence of fatal heart attacks may be explained by the fact that they all occurred early in the study, before the beneficial effects of the vitamin E on the buildup of atherosclerotic plaque had time to occur.

While we await the results from four prospective randomized trials on vitamin E and heart disease, currently under way in Canada, the United States, the United Kingdom, and Italy, I believe there is sufficient strong circumstantial evidence to warrant the taking of 400 to 800 I.U. daily, particularly if you suffer from coronary heart disease. There would not appear to be any harmful side effects, except for people on blood-thinning medications, such as warfarin (Coumadin). Since vitamin E also acts as a mild anticlotting agent, it should not be taken in conjunction with anticoagulants. If in doubt, check with your doctor. Aspirin is also a mild anticlotting agent, but is probably not strong enough to cause a problem for vitamin E takers. Some scientists claim that vitamin E can itself become a toxic oxidizing agent if tissue levels of vitamin C are too low. This seems unlikely if the vitamin E intake is high enough (400–800 I.U.). Alternatively, one can take 250–500 mg of vitamin C along with the vitamin E to obviate this possibility.

The scientific name of vitamin E is tocopherol. It comes in a number of forms, all named after Greek letters, e.g., alpha, beta, gamma, and delta tocopherol. Alpha tocopherol is the most active of these. It occurs naturally, when it is referred to as d-alpha tocopherol, or it can be produced in a synthetic form, known as dl-alpha tocopherol. When you read the label on a container of vitamin E capsules, you will usually find that their strength is stated in International Units (I.Us). This is a measure of biological potency. It so happens that the I.U. standard for vitamin E was set using the synthetic form. Thus, one I.U. of vitamin E equals one milligram of synthetic dl-alpha tocopherol. However, by the same measuring standard, one I.U. equals 1.5 milligrams of the natural d-alpha tocopherol. Since one I.U. is one I.U., whatever the form of vitamin E, you needn't worry if it is natural or synthetic. However, if the strength is expressed in milligrams, then remember that 400 I.Us of potency requires 400 milligrams of dl-alpha tocopherol but only approximately 250 milligrams of d-alpha tocopherol.

If future randomized clinical trials support the results of current retrospective studies, then vitamin E could well play a major role in reducing the incidence of coronary heart disease.

Vitamin C is essential in the manufacture of collagen, the base substance that acts as a cement for many of the tissues and organs of our bodies. It occurs naturally in citrus fruits such as lemons and limes. It was not until 1932 that the specific protective agent in the lime was isolated in the form of vitamin C; two years later, it was synthesized.

While there is good laboratory and biochemical proof that vitamin C is a strong antioxidant, clinical evidence that it lowers the risk of cardiovascular disease is inconclusive. In the Health Professionals' Follow-up Study, it was first reported that men who took a gram of vitamin C daily had a 17% reduction in the incidence of coronary heart disease compared with those who took one-tenth that dose. However, after adjusting for the effects of vitamin E, the benefit of vitamin C disappeared. Two other large studies, one involving 34,000 postmenopausal women and the other 11,000 elderly persons, confirmed this finding. It should be noted, however, that none of these studies looked at a vitamin C–deficient population.

This could be important. One large prospective population study of 1,600 Finnish men over eight years revealed that those who were vitamin C–deficient had as much as three and a half times the risk of a heart attack compared with those who were not. In this context, it should be noted that smoking, alcohol, and high levels of physical stress (such as an exhausting long-distance run) will tend to deplete our vitamin C reserves. One small study has demonstrated that one gram of vitamin C daily could prevent the oxidation of LDL-cholesterol induced by acute cigarette smoking. Thus, there seems a good argument in favor of vitamin C supplementation in populations who are vitamin C–deficient, either because of an inadequate intake of fruit and vegetables, or due to excessive smoking or alcohol intake.

Despite the lack of conclusive evidence in favor of vitamin C supplementation to prevent atherosclerosis, there remains the biochemical justification for its use. As we have seen, vitamin E resides in fatty tissue and protects the fats within the LDL particles from oxidation. Vitamin C is water-soluble and has the potential to protect against water-bound free radicals. It also regenerates vitamin E in its spent form, when it tends to lose its antioxidant effect. On this basis, therefore, it does seem reasonable to take vitamin C as a supplement. Of all the vitamins, vitamin C is probably the cheapest, so cost is not a problem. However, on the matter of safety, there is a cautionary flag.

Vitamin C, normally an antioxidant, can actually promote oxidation when in the presence of excess iron in the tissues. For individuals suffering from hemochromatosis, a genetic but treatable condition in which there is a build-up of iron in the cells of the liver and heart, megadoses of vitamin C can be dangerous because they convert the iron stores into a powerful oxidant, catalytic iron. Some 11% of Caucasians and 8% of Afro-Americans carry the gene for hemochromatosis, so the danger is not insignificant. Most individuals will know if they have the condition, but before taking megavitamin C supplementation, some of us might want to have our iron status measured. Apart from that, there seems little harm, and there could be considerable benefit, in taking from one-half to a gram of vitamin C daily, particularly if you are a smoker, or are not getting your five daily servings of fruit and vegetables.

Beta-carotene is only one of a large number of substances called carotenoids which have been identified in fruits (oranges, tomatoes, cantaloupe, pink grapefruit) and vegetables (carrots, broccoli, brussels sprouts, yellow corn, sweet potatoes). Two large studies, one American (the Health Professionals' Follow-up Study), the other European (the European Community Multicentre Study on Antioxidants, Myocardial Infarction, and Breast Cancer) have demonstrated the benefit of a diet high in total carotenoids in reducing the incidence of coronary disease—but only in current or past smokers. However, this led to several long-term clinical trials to test the health effects of dietary supplementation with one of the best known carotenoids and a proven antioxidant, beta-carotene. The results have not been quite as expected.

A Finnish study (the Alpha-Tocopherol Beta-Carotene Lung Cancer Prevention Study) published in 1994, found that beta-carotene *increased* the risk of lung cancer in smokers, and that men taking the supplement had a higher mortality from heart disease than those taking placebo. Another study, known as CARET (Beta-Carotene and Retinol Efficacy Trial) tested the effect of supplementation on smokers, former smokers, and workers exposed to asbestos. The trial was stopped halfway through its four-year follow-up, because those taking beta-carotene had a *higher* lung cancer rate, and a 26% *greater* incidence of death from coronary disease. Finally, the Physicians' Health Study, which observed the effect of taking 50 milligrams of beta-carotene on alternate days over a 12-year period (the longest trial of beta-carotene to date) by 22,000 American male doctors, found no benefit whatsoever in reducing fatal or nonfatal heart attacks. Obviously we are faced with contradictory findings here. Low levels of beta-carotene in the tissues are associated with increased risk of heart disease; by the same token, high levels appear to be protective. Furthermore, a *diet* high in carotenoids, which includes beta-carotene, increases their content in the body, and contributes to the protective effect from cancer. Supplementation with beta-carotene by itself, however, appears at best to be ineffective, and at worst harmful. How can we explain this? There is no ready answer. It may be that one or more of the other 600 known carotenoids contained in a diet high in fruit and vegetables are the true heart disease protectors, and that loading the body with excessive amounts of beta-carotene prevents their absorption through the gut, or in some way neutralizes their potency. In the meantime, until we solve the mystery, my recommendation would be (i) if you smoke, don't take beta-carotene in supplement form; (ii) get your carotenoids in the form of fruit and vegetables; and (iii) if you know that your diet is inadequate in terms of carotenoid intake, and you feel you need to take beta-carotene, keep the dosage below 15 milligrams daily. There is, after all, still evidence that beta-carotene deficiency is associated with some precancerous lesions.

Flavonoids occur in vegetables, fruits, tea and red wine. They belong to a class of substances called polyphenols and are powerful antioxidants. One large European study of the elderly showed an inverse relationship between flavonoid intake, particularly from tea, onions, and apples, and the incidence of nonfatal and fatal heart attacks. The high content of flavonoids in red wine is said to reduce the oxidation of LDL-cholesterol and explain the so-called French paradox: in France, there is a high intake of dietary fat but a low incidence of coronary heart disease. So, a glass of red wine a day seems like a good idea. However, remember that alcohol can also raise your blood pressure and thereby increase your chance of a stroke. Excessive alcohol consumption can also harm heart muscle, leading to a condition known as cardiomyopathy, which can be associated with sudden death.

Ubiquinone, also known as *coenzyme Q10*, or vitamin Q (although not internationally recognized as a vitamin), was first isolated from beef heart in 1957. It occurs in many foodstuffs, including soybean oil, ocean fish, grains, and nuts. Since then it has attracted increasing interest for its antioxidant properties, estimated experimentally to be ten times stronger than vitamin E. In fact, a number of investigators have found that vitamin E and vitamin Q are interrelated, the latter acting as a kind of catalyst for the former, and also exerting a protective effect. Vitamin Q has also been shown to be of some help in patients suffering from heart failure, although the data are not firm enough and the mechanism for its action insufficiently understood to warrant its routine use in this condition.

A finding possibly of greater interest has been independently described by scientists from the United States and Italy. Both report that treatment with lovastatin, simvastatin, and pravastatin of hypercholesterolemic patients, results in a reduction in vitamin Q blood levels. The significance of this remains uncertain, even assuming that these findings are reproduced by other workers.

There is also the suggestion that vitamin Q exerts a protective effect on heart muscle, and may be of value in the treatment of angina as well as heart failure, or during surgical procedures such as coronary artery bypass grafting or heart transplantation. However, at the moment, treatment with vitamin Q remains outside the mainstream of accepted therapy for coronary artery disease.

Dietary Fiber

Dr. Dennis Burkitt first drew attention to the benefits of fiber in the diet while working as a medical missionary in Africa. He noted that disorders such as gallstones, bowel cancer, hypertension, and coronary heart disease were extremely rare among his African patients, and he came to the conclusion that their absence was due to the fact that the African diet contained a high amount of indigestible roughage, in the form of unmilled grains and cereals, or fiber. Over the past hundred years, this roughage has been gradually processed out of the Western diet. The effect of this lack of fiber in food is to reduce the bulk of the fecal stools and to increase the time of its passage through the intestine. Dr. Burkitt felt that the fiber in the intestine helped the body to excrete cholesterol through the bowel, and this contributed to the low blood cholesterol levels and consequent rarity of coronary artery disease.

Since Dr. Burkitt introduced his theory in the early 1970s, it has been widely accepted by the public and enthusiastically embraced by breakfast cereal manufacturers, who now vie with each other to produce a product with the highest fiber content. There was some disappointment, however, when controlled feeding studies carried out in hospital metabolic wards failed to show that dietary fiber had a cholesterol-lowering effect. There was good evidence that it benefited intestinal problems, but none that it could reduce the incidence of coronary heart disease significantly by altering cholesterol levels.

The matter remained in abeyance for a time, but then came to the fore again when it was realized that dietary fiber exists in a soluble and an insoluble form. Insoluble fiber is found largely in wheat, corn, and rice bran, as well as whole grains and nuts. When in the gut, it absorbs water and, because it is indigestible, cannot pass through the gut wall. Instead it forms a large bulky stool that is easily gripped by the muscular intestinal wall and quickly passes through the alimentary tract. The inclusion of insoluble fiber in the diet is considered beneficial in preventing some bowel diseases, possibly even bowel cancer.

Soluble fiber occurs as pectin in fruits such as apples, pears, oranges, grapefruit, and bananas; as glucan in oats and oat bran, bran cereals, whole grain breads, whole wheat spaghetti, peas, and beans; and as psyllium (sold commercially as the bulk laxative Metamucil), from the seed husk of the plantago, a grain grown in India. These fibers dissolve in water and form a gel in the gut. It was claimed that they could exert a cholesterol-lowering effect. Predictably, there was a surge of products onto the market containing soluble fiber, in particular oat bran.

One of the major proponents of oat bran as a cholesterol-lowerer is Dr. James Anderson of the University of Kentucky. He reported reductions in the order of 15% in cholesterol as a result of adding 50 grams (about a cupful) of oat bran to the diet of a group of hypercholesterolemic subjects. However, a well-designed randomized study from the Harvard Medical School concluded that oat bran achieved its cholesterol-lowering effect not directly, but because it replaced saturated fat in the diet. After all, a large bowl of oat bran in the morning doesn't leave very much room for bacon and eggs. The investigators maintained that replacement of dietary saturated fat by any natural grain or carbohydrate would have the same effect, and that alone, without the addition of oat bran, would be equally effective in lowering cholesterol.

However, let us look at it in perspective. If oat bran works by helping you avoid saturated fat, why not use it? There is no evidence that it can do you any harm. And, as we have seen, there is every reason to believe that insoluble fiber prevents constipation and hemorrhoids, and possibly also diverticulitis and even bowel cancer. In any event, the story isn't quite over yet. A group from the Chicago Center for Clinical Research investigated the hypocholesterolemic effects of the glucan in oat bran. Oat bran, although similar calorically to oatmeal, contains more of the soluble fiber glucan than oatmeal. The researchers took a group of 156 adults who already had high levels of blood cholesterol and also suffered from multiple risk factors for heart disease. They were randomized into three groups. For six weeks, one received supplements of oatmeal, the second oat bran, and the third a placebo. In addition, all were placed on a diet with the same number of calories and the same amount of saturated fat. At the end of the experiment, the placebo group, as might be expected, had no change in cholesterol levels. Supplementation with 2 ounces (57 grams) of oat bran resulted in a 16% drop in LDL-cholesterol, whereas 3 ounces (85 grams) of oatmeal was required to produce an 11.5% reduction. Finally, after a further six weeks' "wash out" during which supplementation was withheld, cholesterol levels returned to their pre-experiment values. The implication here is that the soluble fiber does indeed lower blood cholesterol. Of course, further randomized trials are necessary in order to see what the long-term effect of oat bran supplementation would be.

Psyllium, taken in the form of Metamucil in doses of one rounded teaspoon in an 8-ounce glass of water once or twice a day, has also been shown to reduce cholesterol by approximately 5%. Higher doses may have a greater effect, but recently there have been reports of individuals developing severe allergic reactions to Metamucil. Although such cases are rare, care should be taken if using it for the first time.

The more general complaints of first-time users of any of the dietary fibers are gas and bloating. These can usually be avoided if you increase your fiber intake gradually. Under normal circumstances you probably don't require more than 2 ounces (57 grams) daily.

Currently, North Americans consume one-third to one-half an ounce (about 10 to 14 grams) of fiber a day. The American Dietary Association and the National Cancer Institute recommend 1 ounce (28 grams) of fiber a day, one-third of which should be soluble fiber.

Before leaving the topic, I should emphasize that the overall effect of dietary fiber on blood cholesterol is relatively modest. *Hypercholesterolemia is primarily associated with eating too much saturated fat, not from eating too little fiber.* The place for fiber is as a supplement to a low-fat diet. Remember too that hydrogenated vegetable oil acts as a saturated fat, whether or not it is combined with fiber. There is little point in buying commercially prepared oat bran muffins that include in their list of ingredients a hefty quantity of fully hydrogenated oil.

Fish Oils
During the early 1970s, Danish medical scientist Dr. Jorn Dyerberg investigated reports that Greenland Inuit had only about one-tenth the incidence of heart attacks that their Danish counterparts had. Since Inuit people who had migrated to Denmark lost this immunity, the protective factor seemed more likely environmental than genetic. A careful study of the Inuit lifestyle identified their diet as containing the protective factor. In Greenland, the Inuit diet is largely composed of cold water ocean fish. These creatures contain an oil that is high in two polyunsaturated fatty acids, eicosapentaenoic acid and docosahexaenoic acid. They are also referred to as the Omega-3 fatty acids. Over the past 20 years, considerable research has been carried out on the omega-3s. They appear to benefit the cardiovascular system not so much by altering blood fats (although they do lower blood triglyceride levels), but rather by reducing the tendency of blood to clot within the coronary arteries. This benefit would explain the reduced incidence of heart attack deaths not only in the Greenland Inuit, but also the Japanese, whose diet contains

an average per capita consumption of 3.5 ounces (100 grams) of fish per day.

For most of us, the best way to increase our intake of omega-3 fatty acids is to include a meal of cold water fish in our diet two or more times weekly. In fact, eating fish even once or twice a week may protect us from coronary disease, as a 20-year follow-up of the inhabitants of the small town of Zutphen in the Netherlands has shown. Among those who averaged as little as 7 ounces (200 grams) of fish weekly there were two and a half times fewer deaths from heart attacks than among non-fish eaters. The major sources of omega-3 are anchovies, herring, mackerel, salmon, sardines, tuna, and white fish. As a rule, the darker the flesh of the fish, the higher the omega-3 content. The canned variety is quite suitable, since the fish oil is in the meat. However, don't be fooled by the oil in which it is canned. In the case of sardines and tuna, this is often a vegetable, not an omega-3, oil.

Capsules containing concentrated eicosapentaenoic and docosahexaenoic oils have now appeared on the market and are variously recommended for the prevention of heart disease, hypertension, rheumatoid arthritis, and even migraine headaches. Although there is some experimental evidence to suggest that the omega-3s can be of value in these conditions, you should not take these preparations before discussing it with your physician; they can have unwanted effects. For instance, although they may prevent blood clotting, by the same token they will increase the tendency to bleed excessively from minor cuts or scrapes, tooth extraction, or surgery. In susceptible individuals, or in those who are also taking aspirin as a blood thinner, this effect can be exaggerated. In diabetics, high doses of eicosapentaenoic oils can increase blood sugar levels and interfere with the action of insulin. Better by far, then, to get your omega-3 oils the natural way— from fish.

Olive Oil

Ancel Keys found that monounsaturated fatty acid was neutral, whereas polyunsaturated fatty acid lowered cholesterol. This led to the recommendation that the latter be the preferred substitute for the saturated fatty acids in the diet. However, the commonest source of monounsaturated acid is olive oil, a major component of the Mediterranean diet for thousands of years. Since heart disease is less common in Mediterranean than Northern European countries, the feeling grew that olive oil must have something more to contribute than merely being neutral. This view seemed to be substantiated by a number of studies that suggested that, unlike the vegetable oils, which not only lower total cholesterol but may also reduce HDL-C, olive oil has no such undesirable effect on HDL-C. However, other reports have failed to confirm this. The jury is still out. On the basis that it has certainly stood the test of time, olive oil would not appear to have any harmful effects, but there is no strong scientific basis for preferring it over the vegetable oil linoleic acid as a substitute for saturated fatty acids. Its main benefit may be that it substitutes for animal fats in the Mediterranean diet.

ENDOTHELIUM AND ARGININE

You will recall that in an earlier chapter I described the endothelium as a smooth surface that lines the coronary arteries, permits the uninterrupted flow of blood, and acts as a barrier to the passage of cholesterol particles into the blood vessel wall. Well, in fact, it does all these things, but since the 1980s and largely due to the pioneering work of Dr. Robert Furchgott of New York, we have come to realize that endothelium is a very important part of the coronary vessel wall and that it plays a critical role in the cause and possibly in the treatment of coronary heart disease. In 1986, Dr. Furchgott reported that the endothelium is capable of producing a "relaxing factor," a substance that causes the coronary vessel to dilate and increase blood flow to the heart muscle. A year later, Dr. Salvador Moncado and his team in England identified that substance as nitric oxide, and went on to demonstrate that it is manufactured by the endothelial cells from an amino acid known as L-arginine in response to the mechanical effect of blood flow. When the blood flows quickly through the coronary vessel it tends to flatten the endothelial cells, and this is the stimulus for the cells to convert the L-arginine to nitric oxide, which in turn dilates the vessel and thus permits a greater flow.

What has this to do with the development of atherosclerosis? Animal studies have shown that when the endothelium is damaged (as it could be, for example, by cigarette smoke, the effects of chronic high blood pressure, oxidized LDL-C, high concentrations of homocysteine, or bacteria such as chlamydia), it loses its ability to generate nitric oxide. Instead of dilating in response to an increase in blood flow, it contracts, thereby reducing instead of improving blood supply to heart muscle. Lack of nitric oxide also allows clot to form on the damaged endothelial cells, and generally promotes the development of the atherosclerotic plaque. In the 1990s, animal studies demonstrated that supplementation with L-arginine could restore nitric oxide production, and even retard the development of atherosclerosis in cholesterol-fed rabbits. This suggests that L-arginine could be a new and exciting agent to prevent or treat coronary artery disease in humans. The precise dosage and the trade-off in terms of possible side effects remain to be determined, but the data so far seem quite promising.

6. Detection and Treatment of Coronary Heart Disease

The classic symptoms and signs of angina pectoris and of a heart attack are well known. Any patient who arrives at a doctor's office or an emergency department of a hospital with these symptoms is usually swiftly diagnosed. However, various tests are needed to confirm the diagnosis, particularly when the symptoms are not typical.

The Electrocardiogram
The ECG (or, in America, the EKG) is the most frequently used cardiac diagnostic test. It consists of a tracing of the minute amounts of electrical activity generated by the heart muscle when it contracts. Electrodes, small metal plates, are placed on the body to record the electrical current from different parts of the heart. Usually there are ten electrodes, one over each wrist and above each ankle, and six placed across the front of the chest. These give us an electrical picture of the beating heart as viewed from its front, back, and bottom surface. For convenience, each deflection, or wave, of the tracing is labelled by the consecutive letters P, Q, R, S, and T (Figure 23). The first

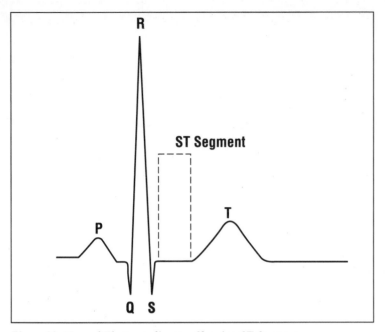

Figure 23: Normal Electrocardiogram Showing ST Segment

deflection, the P wave, is caused by the upper chambers of the heart, the atria, contracting. Thereafter, there is a short pause while the current passes to the lower chambers, the ventricles. When the ventricles contract, they give rise to the QRS wave or complex. After another delay, there is a further flow of current, which recharges the heart and prepares it for its next beat; the recharge results in the T wave. The interval between the end of the QRS complex and the beginning of the T wave is referred to as the ST segment and is very important in modern cardiology. If the shape, particularly the angle, of its slope changes during exercise when the heart is beating rapidly, it can be a very early sign of coronary artery disease.

A heart attack gives rise to characteristic abnormalities in the ECG tracing. These changes may take some hours to develop after the onset of symptoms, but usually they are easily recognizable, even in their early stages. The part of the heart that has been damaged by the attack can be identified by the electrode or group of electrodes showing the greatest abnormalities. Heart attack ECG changes are generally permanent, since the scar tissue, although it functions satisfactorily, never regains the normal pattern of electrical activity. Anginal pain, since it does not cause permanent damage to heart muscle cells, can be detected on the ECG only at the time of the attack, and even then not consistently.

The Exercise Test

We have seen that a person can suffer from coronary artery disease for many years before developing angina. Since anginal symptoms are frequently brought on by exercise, recognition of the disease is delayed even further if the person never exercises. By the time the usual low-level activities of daily living give rise to symptoms, the degree of coronary atherosclerosis is usually quite severe. However, if we can have the subject exercise at gradually increasing intensities of effort, as in an exercise test, we may be able to induce typical anginal pain even when the degree of coronary narrowing is quite moderate and the presence of disease otherwise unrecognized. The exercise test is usually performed on a treadmill or a stationary cycle. The subject is connected to an electrocardiogram, so that a continuous ECG tracing is obtained throughout the test. The speed of the treadmill belt at the start of the test is quite slow, about 2 miles (3 kilometers) per hour. The slope is set at zero. Every two or three minutes, the speed and slope are increased slightly. The initial stages call for a slow easy stroll, gradually progressing to vigorous uphill jogging. If the cycle is used, the level of effort is increased every minute by adjusting the pedal resistance. The test is supervised, or in the case of the Toronto Centre actually carried out, by a physician, assisted by nursing and exercise laboratory staff. The person exercises until forced to stop because of extreme leg fatigue and breath-lessness. The length of time of the test may vary from nine to fifteen minutes, depending on the subject's fitness level. In the case of a coronary patient, the test is sometimes stopped by the physician because of the onset of angina. In this situation, a test is referred to as being a "symptom limited maximal test."

However, the exercise test's major contribution to the early diagnosis of coronary disease comes not just from the detection of anginal pain, but from the fact that it allows us to see changes that occur in the simultaneously recorded exercise ECG *before* the onset of angina. Indeed, these changes may even take place in the *absence* of anginal pain, in which case they are referred to as "silent angina" or, in medical language, silent "ischemia." The abnormalities referred to involve the ST segment. This part of the tracing becomes increasingly depressed as the blood flow through the coronary arteries becomes more restricted (Figure 24). When a coronary-prone patient develops exercise chest pain of uncertain origin accompanied by ST segment depression, we can be almost completely certain that this pain is due to coronary disease. The earlier in the test, and therefore the lower the level of effort at which the pain and/or the ST segment changes occur, the more severe the degree of coronary narrowing. Of course, no medical test is 100% accurate. There are rare occasions when ST depression is due to some other cause (for example, the drug digitalis, or abnormal electrical pathways in the heart, situations with which the physician will be thoroughly familiar). Nevertheless, a positive exercise test in a patient with a strong family history of coronary disease or one who possesses two or more coronary risk factors usually indicates the presence of atherosclerosis.

In addition to ST segment changes, the exercise ECG can also detect the presence of effort-induced irregular heartbeats, which, if they become too frequent, can be

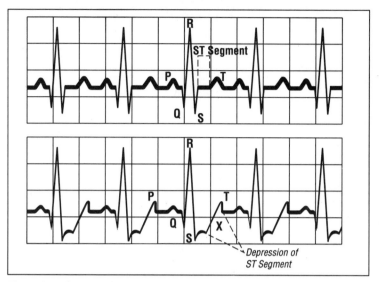

Figure 24: Electrocardiogram Indicating Coronary Disease
(A) Normal electrocardiogram at rest, and (B) showing depression of ST segment during exercise indicating restriction of blood flow through the coronary arteries.

another indication to halt the test. Blood pressure is also monitored every two minutes to see that it is responding normally to exercise. Finally, we can collect and analyze the subject's expired breath throughout the test. This enables us to measure the amount of oxygen being used at peak effort, giving us the maximum oxygen intake, or VO$_2$max, an excellent measure of cardiovascular fitness. From this we can calculate a safe and effective exercise training intensity. Furthermore, using the information obtained from this analysis, we can construct a graph showing how the breathing rate increases with each stage of the test. We will then be able to see the point at which the subject's breathing starts to become more rapid and labored. This point signifies the early onset of fatigue and lactic acid build-up and is referred to as the anaerobic threshold (Figure 25). It corresponds to about 60% of the peak oxygen intake, and a level of 12 to 14 on the Borg Scale of Perceived Exertion (Figure 34), and is a further

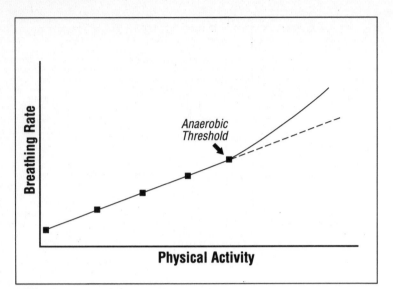

Figure 25: Anaerobic Threshold
The anaerobic threshold is the point at which the relationship between breathing and exercise becomes non-linear. This is an appropriate level of exertion for endurance training.

corroboration of the correct training intensity. Collection of expired air is carried out through a mask connected by flexible hosing to a sophisticated machine that analyzes the breath for oxygen and carbon dioxide content. Since cardiac departments are more interested in detecting coronary disease than in prescribing exercise, they usually dispense with this equipment. However, it has been used in assessing our patients at the Toronto Centre since the program started in 1968.

OTHER METHODS OF INVESTIGATING
THE HEART

Echocardiography

High-frequency sound waves are generated by an ultra-sonic machine and are "bounced" off the heart; these sound echoes are then converted into electrical energy to display a moving image on an oscilloscope screen. Thus, one can determine the size of the heart's chambers, the thickness of its walls, and the efficiency of its performance. If the examination is done before and immediately after exercise, one is even better able to detect abnormalities in the heart's pumping capacity. There is no radioactivity involved, and the patient feels nothing during the examination.

Radionuclide Imaging

This procedure involves the use of radioactive substances called radio isotopes, which are injected into the bloodstream through a vein in the arm and then detected in the body by a highly sensitive Gamma camera. Two types of tests are in common use. In the first, radionuclide ventriculography, the isotope (technetium-99) is attached to the red cells, and pictures are taken of the blood pool within the chambers of the heart, particularly the ventricles. The amount of blood ejected with each beat can be seen, as well as the movement of the walls of the heart, and the pumping efficiency assessed accordingly. In the second, the isotope (thallium-201 or a similar substance) is injected into the vein and is then carried through the coronary arteries to the walls of the heart. If blood flow is reduced in a particular coronary artery branch because of atherosclerotic narrowing, the camera will show little or no radionuclide material in the portion of the wall supplied by the narrowed artery. This type of imaging is usually combined with an exercise test, which accentuates its effect and can be helpful in diagnosing doubtful cases of effort-induced angina or ST segment depression. The radio isotopes used in these tests have very short half-lives, which means they are cleared very rapidly from the body. They are also used in such minute quantities that they do not constitute any danger to the patient.

Telemetry
This test consists of radio transmission of the ECG to a receiver-printer. It permits an ECG in situations where solid wire connecting cables between the patient and the ECG machine would be impractical, for example, when the patient is walking or jogging. In the cardiac rehabilitation setting, it is used to monitor patients for the presence of exercise-induced ST segment depression or skipped beats, usually during workouts or simulated job tasks. It is also used to check the patient's ability to take a pulse accurately. The transmission range is usually up to 110 yards (100 meters), provided there are no obstructions between the patient and the receiver.

Ambulatory Electrocardiogram Monitoring
This technique is used to detect ECG abnormalities that are suspected to be occurring during activities of daily living and while away from the hospital or doctor's office. Chest electrodes are connected to a small tape recorder that is strapped to the waist. The apparatus is usually worn for 24 hours, during which time the patient keeps an activity diary, recording any unusual symptoms. When the tape is returned, it is run through a computerized rapid analyzer, which detects any irregularities and relates them to the comments on the diary.

Coronary Angiography
Unlike the previous tests, this one is "invasive." A thin hollow tube, or catheter, is carefully pushed through a small

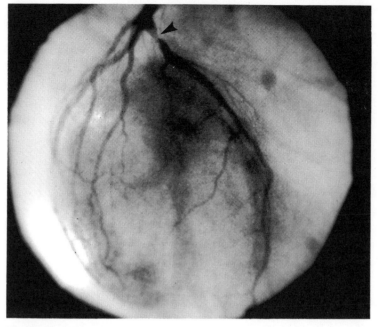

Figure 26: Angiogram
An angiogram X-ray of coronary arteries showing narrowing (see arrow) in the upper portion of the anterior descending branch of the left coronary artery.

cut in a groin or arm artery and then threaded up the artery into the aorta until its tip lies opposite the openings of the coronary arteries. The procedure is carried out by a cardiologist, who carefully watches the passage of the catheter on an X-ray display. Once the tip of the catheter is in position, a dye that is visible on the X-ray is injected into all three coronary arteries and its flow observed on a large video screen; the pictures are also recorded on film for subsequent playback and re-examination (Figure 26). As the dye passes down the coronary arteries, one can see any narrowing or obstruction. The procedure causes only minor discomfort (a hot "flush" as the dye is being injected), but the patient has to keep the affected leg or arm still for about six hours after the procedure so as to prevent bleeding from the incision. Nowadays there is an increasing tendency for cardiac catheterization to be carried out on an outpatient basis.

The risks of catheterization are minimal, but the most serious includes precipitating a fatal heart attack or a stroke. While the chances of this are only about one in a thousand or even less, catheterization is not carried out except in situations where angioplasty or coronary artery bypass surgery is being seriously considered, or to help in the diagnosis where there is uncertainty as to the cause of severe chest pain or an abnormal exercise test. Certainly mere curiosity as to the degree of coronary disease is not a usual indication.

MEDICATIONS FREQUENTLY USED IN THE TREATMENT OF CORONARY DISEASE

There are a number of drugs used in the treatment of coronary heart disease. The commonest groups are discussed here.

Nitrates

This group of drugs is used to treat angina. They act by opening up, or dilating, the veins and arteries (including the coronaries) throughout the body, thus reducing the work load on the heart and improving its blood supply. They come in a number of preparations. The short-acting nitroglycerine tablet is placed under the tongue until it dissolves; its effect is lost if it is swallowed. It relieves anginal pain quickly, usually within a minute or so, and the relief lasts for up to an hour. It can cause a throbbing headache, or even fainting in some people. These side effects lessen with use. It can also prevent angina if taken before exercise.

Nitroglycerine tablets deteriorate with time and should be replaced after about two months. Their strength declines more rapidly if they are stored in a plastic container with cotton batting. Better to keep them in a glass bottle with a foil-lined cap.

Nitroglycerine aerosol sprays are now in common use, the usual dose being one or two puffs. Adhesive skin patches are yet another form of delivering the drug. They are usually applied over the chest and are intended to maintain a constant level of nitroglycerine in the blood. However, it has been established that tolerance, with loss of anti-anginal effect, can develop with continuous nitrate administration. Apparently this is prevented by intermittent use. Therefore, if patches are used, they are generally removed for a time during a 24-hour period, usually during the night.

Long-acting nitrate is given in the form of isosorbide dinitrate (trade name Isordil); unlike the nitroglycerine tablet, it is not destroyed by the internal digestive juices, so it can be swallowed. The anti-anginal effect lasts four to six hours and may be prescribed three or four times a day.

Beta-Adrenoreceptor-Blocker (Beta-Blockers)

The increase in heart rate and blood pressure that accompanies the body's "fight or flight" response is brought about by the action of the hormones adrenaline and noradrenaline on small, button-like structures, called beta-adrenoreceptors, that are located throughout the heart muscle and in the walls of the blood vessels. Beta-blockers prevent or block the entry of these hormones into the receptors and so cancel out their stimulating effect. Thus, they reduce the speed and force of the heartbeat, that is, the pulse rate and blood pressure. Beta-blockers are used in the treatment of the following conditions: (i) exercise- or stress-induced angina, because they reduce the work of the heart; (ii) hypertension, because they reduce blood pressure; (iii) certain types of irregular heartbeats (skipped beats); (iv) heart attack, in order to prevent a later fatal or nonfatal recurrence; (v) glaucoma, in the form of eye drops, because they lower the pressure inside the eye; (vi) migraine, because they prevent the blood vessels in the brain from overdilating; and (vii) occasionally to calm nerves or tremor (by lowering adrenaline levels) in public speakers or actors on "first nights," or professional sportsmen such as marksmen or pool players (their use in competition is banned!).

There are a few real contraindications to the use of beta-blockers. They may not be suitable for patients suffering from severe asthma, bronchitis, or other forms of lung disease, because they block the beta-receptors in the lungs that, as part of the noradrenaline effect, open up the airways so as to receive more oxygen. They are also not good for patients who suffer from peripheral vascular disease, in which atherosclerosis has reduced the circulation of blood to the legs, because they can cause cold feet and hands. They can also interfere with glucose metabolism and are used only with caution in insulin-dependent diabetics.

Although small doses of a beta-blocker may not affect heart rate, larger doses invariably will, and allowance must be made for this when using pulse rates as a guide in exercise training. This will be dealt with more fully in Chapter 12.

Some beta-blockers in large doses may hinder full utilization by the skeletal muscle of its major fuels, fat and starch, and in this way cause early muscle fatigue. The exerciser may suddenly become tired during a workout and have to stop because of leg fatigue. Where this problem is excessive, improvement may be obtained by switching to another beta-blocker, one that has less peripheral effect. Other side effects may include diarrhea, nausea, depression, loss of sexual urge, and reduction of HDL-cholesterol.

Finally, beta-blockers should not be stopped suddenly

after they have been used for a prolonged period of time. This can result in a sudden over-sensitivity to noradrenaline, with consequent swift return of symptoms such as severe angina or marked elevation of blood pressure. There have even been reports of heart attacks occurring after sudden cessation of a beta-blocker. Where the medication has to be stopped, it should be done gradually and under the supervision of your physician.

Since they were first introduced in 1956, many new beta-blockers have been developed. They differ from each other only insofar as they may act primarily to relieve angina, or lower blood pressure, or both, or in whether they are long- or short-acting, or in the manner in which they bring about various minor side effects in different individuals. The choice can be made only by the physician. The most commonly prescribed go under the trade names of propranolol (Inderal), timolol (Blocadren), nadolol (Corgard), sotalol (Sotacor), acebutolol (Sectral), atenolol (Tenormin), metoprolol (Lopressor), pindolol (Visken), and amiodarone (Cordarone).

Calcium Channel Blockers

This class of heart drug was introduced in 1976 and was approved for use in heart disease in North America in the 1980s. It acts by slowing the rate at which calcium moves backwards and forwards across the walls of the cells via special passages called calcium channels. Slowing the passage of calcium reduces the force with which the cells work. The effect on heart muscle cells is to lessen the force and speed of the heart's contractions, thus reducing cardiac work load. The arteries of the body, including the coronary arteries, respond to the calcium channel blockers by relaxing. Calcium channel blockers are therefore used to treat angina and also hypertension. Because they relax the muscular walls of the coronary arteries, they are unique in their ability to treat a particular type of angina known as Prinzmetal's angina, which occurs at rest, and is due to a spasm of the coronary arteries. The cause of the condition is unknown; it may even occur in those whose coronary arteries are free from atherosclerosis, and, as I have said, until the introduction of the calcium channel blockers, it was a major treatment problem. The most common calcium channel blockers used in North America go under the trade names of verapamil (Isoptin), nicardipine (Cardene), diltiazem (Cardizem), nifedipine (Adalat), and amlodipine (Norvasc). Each has a slightly different action, and, as with the beta-blockers, your physician will choose whichever is most suitable in your case.

Digitalis
Derived originally from the leaf of the common purple foxglove, digitalis, or digoxin, was first used by an English general practitioner, Dr. William Witherspoon, in the 1700s. He administered it to his heart disease patients in the form of a tea, and obtained almost immediate relief of their symptoms. It has been used by physicians ever since in the treatment of heart failure and also in a form of heart irregularity called atrial fibrillation. Digitalis tends to slow the resting heart rate. It can also produce a form of ST segment depression (see page 142), seen at rest and during an exercise test, which is perfectly harmless but if not recognized as such can give the impression that the patient is suffering from restricted coronary blood flow.

DRUGS THAT REDUCE THE ABILITY OF THE BLOOD TO CLOT

PLATELET INHIBITORS

Aspirin
In its natural form, salicylic acid, aspirin is obtained from the bark of various species of the willow and poplar.

Today it is used in its synthesized form, acetylsalicylic acid. The humble aspirin has been used by physicians since the days of ancient Greece. It is still used extensively to reduce fever, relieve pain, reduce inflammation, and treat arthritis. It leapt into prominence in the context of coronary heart disease when it was discovered that it was a mild anticlotting agent. It acts by inhibiting the first steps in the formation of a blood clot, which is the clumping together of the blood platelet cells and then the sticking of these clumps to the inner wall of an artery. Since this process is often the first stage in the development of a heart attack, this discovery led to a series of clinical trials to determine if aspirin could (i) reduce the death rate from a heart attack in its early stages shortly after the onset of pain; (ii) reduce the likelihood of a recurrent heart attack; (iii) reduce the likelihood of a future heart attack in patients suffering from severe angina; and (iv) prevent a first heart attack in healthy individuals who are apparently free from coronary disease.

The answer given by the various studies to the first three questions is an absolute and unqualified yes.

Obviously, in these situations, aspirin is given by prescription and at the discretion of the patient's physician. The latter will take into account the fact that aspirin does, however, have some undesirable side effects. It is a well-known gastric irritant and can lead to peptic ulcers or cause them to bleed. People with a strong family or personal history of hemorrhagic stroke (a type caused by a blood vessel bursting and bleeding into the brain tissue) probably should not take aspirin at all.

What about the use of aspirin in healthy individuals in order to protect them from heart disease? In essence, we have two studies, one American and one British, which appear to contradict one another. The American study involved 22,000 male physicians. Half were assigned to take one 325-mg aspirin tablet every other

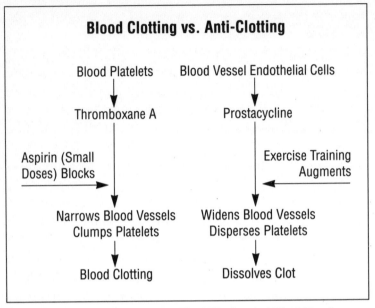

Figure 27: The Interaction Between Blood Platelets and Blood Vessel Endothelial Cells in Blood Clot Formation

day, while the other half were given an aspirin-free placebo. At the end of five years, it was found that the aspirin takers had about 45% fewer heart attacks than the non–aspirin takers. The British study, smaller in size and using a higher dose of aspirin (500 mg daily), found no advantage in terms of fatal or nonfatal heart attacks to the aspirin takers.

What can we make of this? Firstly, there is the question of dosage. The American trial used a 325-mg tablet every other day, whereas the British study used 500 mg every day. It could be that the higher doses of aspirin block not only the action of thromboxane A, which causes platelets to clump together, but also the formation of prostacycline, the substance produced by the endothelium, which prevents the platelets from sticking to one another and to the blood vessel wall (Figure 27).

Also, the greatest decrease in heart attacks occurred in

the American physicians aged 50 years and older; there was no difference in the number of heart attacks in those under the age of 50, whether or not they took aspirin. Taking everything into account, however, it does seem that taking a junior aspirin (80 mg) every day or even every second day is probably a good idea; it can probably reduce your risk of a heart attack by about 30%, particularly if you are over the age of 50.

THROMBOLYTICS

These are the latest so-called wonder drugs. Because they dissolve the fibrin strands in the blood clot, they are also referred to as "clot-busters." Administered by intravenous injection within the first few hours after the onset of a heart attack, they break up the clot in the coronary artery, restore normal blood flow, and prevent damage to heart muscle. A number of large-scale international clinical trials have demonstrated that their use, in appropriate cases, reduces the risk of death from heart attack by as much as 50%. The two drugs currently in use are streptokinase and tissue plasminogen activator (TPA).

TPA is of considerable interest, since it is a natural clot-buster produced by the body, and I will refer later to the fact that exercise training enhances its natural effectiveness. It is now manufactured by the process of genetic engineering to give recombinant tissue plasminogen activator (rt-PA) and is commonly used to treat an acute heart attack.

CHOLESTEROL-LOWERING DRUGS

These fall into four broad categories: the statins, the bile resins, the fibrates, and niacin.

The Statins

This new group of drugs suppresses the liver's ability to make cholesterol. The commonest in use are lovastatin (Mevacor), simvastatin (Zocor), pravastatin (Pravachol), atorvastatin (Lipitor) and fluvastatin (Lescol). These are the most powerful cholesterol-lowering drugs available. They are taken with the evening meal, or before going to bed, since cholesterol manufacture takes place mainly during sleeping hours. Studies show that these drugs have relatively few side effects. Very rarely, they can cause damage to the liver and the peripheral muscles, and for this reason the manufacturers advise regular blood tests to check for this, particularly in the early months of treatment. If these side effects do occur, they are readily reversed when the drug is stopped. Both simvastatin and pravastatin have been used in landmark studies in the 1990s, and their effectiveness in reducing fatal heart attacks in patients with coronary heart disease has convinced the medical profession worldwide of the value of cholesterol-lowering therapy. New and improved members of the group will undoubtedly appear in the future.

The Fibrates

The commonest are gemfibrozil (Lopid) and bezafibrate (Lipidil); both come in capsule form and are taken by mouth. These are most effective in reducing triglycerides and increasing HDL-cholesterol levels. In the Helsinki Heart Study (see page 112) in which gemfibrozil was the treatment drug, the major benefits were felt to be due not to the reduction in LDL-cholesterol but rather the large increase in HDL-cholesterol and reduction in triglycerides. A new generation of studies, including one which involves a joint effort between Australia, New Zealand, and Finland, will investigate the possibility that some of the newer fibrates on the market will produce even further reductions in coronary heart disease than those seen with the statins alone.

The Bile Resins

The commonest in use are cholestyramine (Questran) and colestipol (Colestid). These come in the form of granules, either in bulk, or more conveniently, in one-dose packages. They are mixed with water and taken with meals. The resins are not absorbed into the bloodstream but pass unaltered through the gut. Their action is to increase the excretion of bile and cholesterol in the stools. The side effects include gas, bloating, and constipation, but these tend to lessen with continued use. The introduction of the statins has tended to reduce the use of these medications.

Niacin

Otherwise known as vitamin B3, nicotinic acid, or nicotinamide, niacin is found naturally in liver, lean meat, poultry, fish, whole grains, beans, and nuts. In the 1950s, it was found that if it was given in large doses, 1 to 2 grams or more daily, it could dramatically reduce triglycerides and boost HDL cholesterol.

There is an obvious appeal to using a naturally occurring substance such as a vitamin to cure or prevent heart disease. However, vitamins given in megadoses are drugs, and as such can have unpleasant side effects. The fact that they can be bought over the counter in any drugstore or health food store may make them even more of a potential hazard. In doses in excess of 250 milligrams, the side effects of niacin are more irritating than dangerous and include flushing of the skin, tingling, itching, and headache. In most cases, these can be avoided by building up to the larger doses gradually, taking niacin with food, or taking an aspirin an hour or so before the niacin tablet. However, doses of niacin in the order of 1 to 2 grams or more daily can have more serious side effects. Gastric irritation is not uncommon, and peptic ulcers may be aggravated. Blood sugar levels can be increased, which can pose a problem for the very individuals who often suffer from low HDL-cholesterol and high triglycerides, i.e., Type II diabetics. A more serious problem involves the use of the sustained-release or long-acting niacin, which was developed in order to prevent the flushing and tingling that occurred with the short-acting tablet. Unfortunately, it seems that the long-acting form can be more toxic to the liver, and a number of cases have been reported of individuals who have developed liver damage after taking 2 to 4 grams of sustained release niacin daily over a period of months.

Finally, niacin can sometimes cause problems when taken at the same time as other cholesterol-lowering drugs, such as the statins.

Despite all this, niacin remains one of our most potent and consistent HDL-cholesterol boosters, and if you have low HDL-cholesterol readings, it may be a valuable option. However, you should only take it under the direction of your physician. In that way, not only will your cholesterol be monitored every six months or so, but you can also have blood glucose and liver function tests carried out at the same time.

It should be stressed that all these drugs have side effects and should be used only after a trial of low-fat diet, weight reduction, and exercise has failed to reduce elevated cholesterol levels.

DRUGS USED FOR HEART FAILURE AND/OR HYPERTENSION

Diuretics

These are commonly referred to as "water pills"; they help the body to lose excess water and salt by increasing urine flow. This action prevents "waterlogging" of the legs and ankles, as well as the lungs, which occurs as a result of heart failure. The loss of water from the blood also reduces the total blood volume, which in turn causes the pressure to drop in the blood vessels. Thus, diuretics are also used to treat hypertension. Diuretics can have some undesirable side effects, all of which can, fortunately, be prevented easily. One of the most serious is the loss of too much potassium from the body; it passes out in the urine together with the sodium in the salt. Not enough potassium causes weakness and can also trigger irregular heart rhythm in the form of skipped beats. To avoid these, potassium supplements can be taken in the form of potassium pills or fresh fruit and vegetables, which are rich in potassium. Alternatively your doctor can prescribe a special type of potassium-sparing diuretic that does not cause potassium loss. Other side effects include a disturbance in the way the body metabolizes glucose, and therefore diabetes may be a contraindication. Some diuretics given over a prolonged period of time can cause attacks of gout. Finally, they may also increase blood triglycerides and reduce HDL-cholesterol levels; these undesirable changes can, however, be offset by diet and exercise.

There are numerous diuretics on the market, but the most commonly used are hydrochlorothiazide (HydroDiuril, Aldactazide), furosemide (Lasix), chlorthalidone (Hygroton), and triamterene (Dyazide); the last is an example of a "potassium sparer."

Angiotensin-Converting Enzyme (ACE) Inhibitors

First extracted from the venom of a pit viper, this group of drugs prevents the formation in the body of a substance called angiotensin, the action of which is to constrict the arteries. ACE inhibitors allow the blood vessels to dilate, thereby dropping the blood pressure and relieving the load on a heart. These agents are playing an increasingly successful role in treatment of heart disease, and many more are in the development process. The most common in use now are captopril (Capoten), enalapril (Vasotec), lisinopril (Prinivil), losantin (Cozaar), and quinapril (Accupril). Side effects are seldom serious, but the most troublesome is a dry irritating cough, which can lead to changing or discontinuing the drug. ACE inhibitors have emerged as a powerful and very important group of drugs, with the capacity to reduce short- and long-term mortality after a heart attack and vastly improve the outlook of patients suffering from heart failure.

CARDIAC SURGERY AND OTHER PROCEDURES

Coronary Artery Bypass Graft Surgery

In May 1967, Dr. René Favaloro carried out the first coronary artery bypass graft (CABG) procedure on a patient suffering from severe coronary atherosclerosis. Since then, the popularity of the procedure has increased dramatically until it is now a commonplace operation carried out in all the major medical centers throughout the world.

Although technically complex, the operation is simple in concept. Using a length of vein from the patient's leg, or a segment of artery taken from the chest wall (the internal mammary artery), the surgeon bypasses the atherosclerotic narrowing in the coronary artery by stitching (i.e., grafting) one end of the vein or artery onto the base of the aorta and the other into the portion of coronary

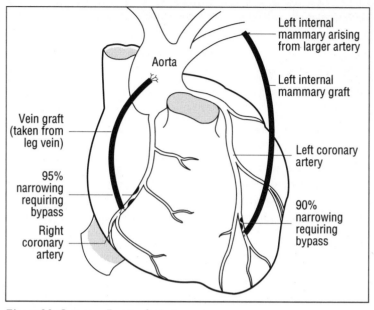

Figure 28: Coronary Bypass Surgery
A vein and an internal mammary artery graft.

artery beyond the narrowing (Figure 28).

Broadly speaking, the benefits of coronary artery bypass graft surgery can be twofold: firstly, an alleviation or abolition of anginal symptoms; and secondly, an improved life expectancy. Is CABG surgery a quick cure-all for coronary artery disease? Only the most naive would come to that conclusion. First of all, there is a risk. Granted it is small, but no surgeon will give you a 100% guarantee that the result will be exactly as you wish. Also, remember that coronary atherosclerosis is a metabolic disease. Fixing the plumbing will neither eliminate the cause nor prevent progression of the disease process. This was brought home dramatically by a report from the Montreal Heart Institute in 1984 of a ten-year follow-up of patients who had undergone CABG surgery. Coronary angiography at the end of that period showed that 29% of the bypass grafts had blocked as a result of atherosclerosis,

33% showed atherosclerotic narrowing, and, even more disturbing, 47% of the previously healthy arteries now showed atherosclerotic narrowing. Admittedly, surgical techniques have improved considerably since then, and there is now more frequent use of the internal mammary artery as a graft; this is a blood vessel located in the muscles of the chest wall that is very resistant to the development of atherosclerosis.

Coronary artery bypass surgery is a more dangerous procedure for women than men. The operative mortality rate is twice as high, 4% compared with 2%. This could be due to the fact that the female patient is older. The operation is also more technically difficult in a woman, because of her smaller coronary arteries. Then again, these results may be biased by preselection. After all, if cardiologists carry out angiography only on those women with the most severe symptoms, then those who undergo surgery are bound to have more extensive coronary disease than their male counterparts and obtain a less successful result. This might also explain why women have less relief of angina after surgery than men and continue to complain more of fatigue and physical incapacity. Nevertheless, once through the operation, their long-term five- and ten-year survival rates appear to be the same as men's.

Recently, the introduction of minimally invasive CABG surgery has generated great interest among surgeons and patients alike. So far it has been practiced on only a few patients, but I have no doubt that within five years it will be a viable alternative to the current procedure, which requires the sternum to be split and the chest to be opened widely, allowing the surgeon to operate on a non-beating heart while the blood is being circulated around the body by a heart-lung machine.

The minimally invasive technique involves making a small 2-inch opening in the chest wall through which the surgeon, using specially designed instruments, isolates

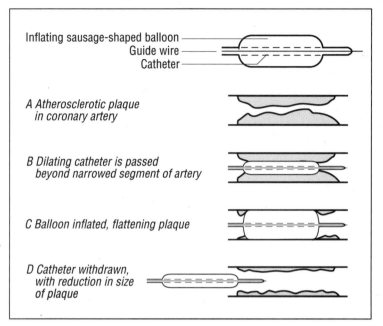

Inflating sausage-shaped balloon
Guide wire
Catheter

A *Atherosclerotic plaque in coronary artery*

B *Dilating catheter is passed beyond narrowed segment of artery*

C *Balloon inflated, flattening plaque*

D *Catheter withdrawn, with reduction in size of plaque*

Figure 29: Percutaneous Transluminal Coronary Angioplasty (PTCA)

the internal mammary artery, and then attaches it to the narrowed coronary artery. The procedure can be carried out while the heart is still beating, although this is technically more difficult and currently suitable only for use in grafting a single vessel, usually the left anterior descending. Alternatively, the heart can be stopped and the blood bypassed through the heart-lung machine by way of catheters passed up to the heart through the arteries in the groins. This procedure, known as port-access cardiopulmonary bypass, also allows the surgeon to carry out multivessel coronary artery grafting without opening the chest.

Angioplasty

Since 1977, there has been an alternative procedure to bypass surgery for certain potential surgical candidates. In that year, Dr. Andreas Gruentzig of Zurich (sadly, killed in a small-airplane accident at the height of his career) performed the first percutaneous transluminal coronary angioplasty (PTCA). A thin catheter, with a distensible balloon at its tip, is inserted into the coronary artery until it reaches the narrowed area. The balloon is then inflated, so as to flatten the atherosclerotic deposit and thus restore normal blood flow (Figure 29). Compared with surgery, PTCA is a relatively minor procedure, not unlike a routine coronary angiogram. There is no surgical scar; the patient is in hospital only overnight and can resume normal activities in two or three days. As with surgery, the major indication for angioplasty is severe effort angina, which is not amenable to routine medical treatment.

Currently, however, some 25% to 30% of angioplasties fail within 6 months, the atherosclerotic narrowing recurs, and the procedure needs to be repeated. Thereafter, the success rate is high. However, the introduction of coronary stents have markedly improved the success rate of angioplasty. Stents are expandable metallic coiled springs or scaffoldings, which are placed on the surface of an angioplasty balloon. The balloon is inflated, the stent is expanded and implanted in the arterial wall; the balloon is then deflated and withdrawn, leaving the scaffolding to hold the vessel open. Stenting has significantly reduced the need for repeat angioplasties. Because the stent is a foreign body, it can give rise to blood clots on its surface, and for this reason the patient is required to take the antiplatelet agents aspirin and ticlopidine (Ticlid), before the procedure, and to continue the ticlopidine for one month afterwards.

There have been conflicting reports on the benefits of angioplasty (PTCA) in women. Some have found a higher recurrence in narrowing rate at 6 and 12 months than in men and more complications occurring during the procedure itself. This has been explained on the basis of smaller arteries, more delicate vessel walls, and particularly in younger women, a more aggressive form of coronary disease. Others have not had the same experience and maintain that complications and recurrence are no more frequent than in men. As in CABG surgery, the long-term results are similar in both men and women.

Heart Transplantation

After some false and shaky starts in the 1970s (due largely to overly optimistic predictions and subsequent bad publicity), the 1980s saw the establishment of a firm foundation for future widespread success of heart transplantation. The discovery of new medications to overcome the major problem of rejection has not only enabled the patient with a new heart to be out of hospital in a matter of weeks, but it has also improved the five-year survival rate to well above 70%. There are now 297 centers in the world performing over 3,000 heart transplants annually. One of the barriers to expanding the service is the lack of donor hearts.

Heart transplantation is carried out when the patient's life is threatened by severe heart failure. Since the commonest cause of failure is extensive coronary disease, fewer younger women are candidates for a heart replacement operation. In fact, the men outnumber the women by about six to one. Although for some reason there is a tendency for women to have more episodes of rejection during the early postsurgical months, this does not affect their short- and long-term survival rate, which is the same as that for the men.

7. Can Physical Activity Prevent Heart Disease?

If time travel were possible, a visitor from a bygone age to the twentieth century would surely be impressed by the extent to which we have eliminated physical activity from our daily routine. Modern transportation methods have made walking almost entirely a leisure activity. The elevator and the escalator save us from climbing steps. Automation is the order of the day in the factory and on the farm. Television and personal computers keep us tied to our chair during the evenings and weekends. As if that weren't enough, we now have golf courses that display the sign "No walking permitted: golfers must use electric carts provided"! The United States Department of Health has estimated that whereas at the turn of the century more than 30% of all the energy expended by the workforce came from muscular effort, this figure had dropped to less than 1% by the mid-twentieth century.

Human beings have been civilized for only the last 10,000 years; for a million years before we discovered that we could grow and eat grain (provided we stayed around long enough to reap it), we were nomads and hunters. We moved with the game, walking, running, stalking, and constantly setting up and breaking camp. Is 10,000 years long enough to extinguish the needs of our bodies for activity and motion? If it were, why is the child still afraid of the dark? Why does our hair stand on end and why do our pupils dilate in preparation for fight or flight when we are startled? We are closer to our Stone Age ancestors than we sometimes choose to admit, so, if we choose to become couch potatoes, we do so at our own risk.

Lessons from Primitive People

Would you like to live to be 100? For years, we have heard tales of communities where centenarians are commonplace; not only that, but they are healthy and alert enough to work until they are in their eighties. Scientists and gerontologists (physicians who specialize in the treatment of the aged) have become particularly interested in these reports. The three regions of the world most renowned for longevity are the Ecuadoran Andes, the Karakoram mountains in Kashmir, and the Abkhazia region of the former southern Soviet Union. On-the-spot research in these areas has verified that ages of 90 to 100 years are not unusual. Heart attacks are extremely rare. Why is this so?

The inhabitants of high Ecuador and Kashmir eat sparingly of a diet low in animal fat; conversely, the Abkhazians eat well, with meat and dairy products as regular items. Smoking is common in all three areas, and most of the old people enjoy their wine, vodka, or local spirit. Researchers have remarked that in all three areas, the lifestyle is characterized by lack of stress, contentment with one's station in life, and heavy involvement of the aged in both family and civic affairs. People expect to live to a ripe old age and assume they will work for as long as they are capable. Any or all of these factors may make important contributions to their longevity. A more objective finding, however, is their high degree of cardiovascular fitness. In all three areas, their work involves heavy physical labor interspersed with a great deal of walking, not infrequently over hilly terrain.

Dr. Alexander Leaf, an American cardiologist who has made a study of these people in their own environment, repeatedly found a high level of endurance fitness in the aged. He was certainly impressed with their capacity for heavy work. He wrote, "Markhti Tarkil...walks half a mile downhill to his daily bath in the river and then climbs uphill again. Surely any day a man can do this he must be too fit to die. The next day he repeats this physical activity and so on, day after day while the years roll by, and at 104, Tarkil is still much too fit to die!" On one occasion, Dr. Leaf toiled up a steep mountainside to interview a 106-year-old shepherd. The journey took him six hours, and the going was so rough that two of the four-man party, including the interpreter, had to turn back. The cardiologist's pride on making it to the top was, however, short-lived; it turned out that the ancient shepherd made the journey regularly in three hours! Dr. Leaf took the lesson to heart: on his return home, he commenced jogging as a hobby.

THE MEDICAL EVIDENCE FOR THE BENEFITS OF EXERCISE IN CORONARY HEART DISEASE

Occupational Physical Activity
In 1953, Professor Jeremy Morris of the British Medical Research Council published an article in the medical journal *The Lancet* entitled "Coronary Heart Disease and Physical Activity at Work." It compared the incidence of heart disease in 31,000 male bus drivers and bus conductors working for the London Transport Department. The drivers were found to suffer one and a half times as many anginal attacks and twice as many fatal and nonfatal heart attacks as the conductors. In his article, Professor Morris suggested that the likeliest explanation for this difference

might lie in the nature of the two jobs. Driving is a sedentary activity requiring minimal expenditure of energy; the conductor, on the other hand, has to collect fares. In a double-decker bus, this activity necessitates an average of 24 trips an hour up and down the winding staircase of the moving vehicle, in addition to walking back and forth along the aisles of the upper and lower compartments. Over an eight-hour shift, the energy expenditure is considerable.

Israel has a high prevalence of heart disease, and its doctors have carried out much excellent research on the topic. Probably the best known to physicians is the work of Dr. Daniel Brunner. In pursuing Morris's findings, Dr. Brunner made use of a unique feature of Israeli life, the existence of kibbutzim. In these communities, people live in a uniform environment, eating the same food, experiencing the same climate, and largely subject to the same external stresses. Obviously, a study carried out in such a setting eliminates many sources of error. In analyzing the cause of death of 10,000 residents of a kibbutz over a period of 15 years, Brunner ascertained that "the incidence of angina, myocardial infarction and fatalities due to ischemic heart disease was found to be *two and a half to four* times greater in sedentary workers than in non-sedentary workers."

In North America, work along similar lines was being carried out by the epidemiologist and physician Professor Ralph Paffenbarger of Berkeley, California. From 1951 through 1972, he studied the incidence of heart disease in some 6,000 longshoremen living in the San Francisco Bay area. This was before the advent of containerization, and he was able to stratify his subjects into light, moderate, and heavy workers. He found that the light workers had two and a half times the incidence of fatal heart attacks and three times the incidence of sudden cardiac death compared with the heavy or moderate physical workers. This benefit persisted even when the ill effects of high blood pressure, obesity, previous heart disease, and cigarette smoking were taken into account. According to Professor Paffenbarger, physical activity reduced the chance of a fatal heart attack by 54%, whereas stopping smoking or reducing high blood pressure cut the risk by only 27% and 29% respectively.

Other investigators reported similar results. Dr. Henry Taylor compared active U.S. railroad switchmen and sedentary ticket clerks; he found the latter had three times higher death rates from heart attacks. Dr. Harold Kahn, also in the United States, and Jeremy Morris, in England, looked at postal workers, comparing mail carriers and sorting clerks; the active carriers had half the heart disease of the sedentary clerks and an even greater protection against sudden cardiac death.

Leisure-time Exercise
As physical work became increasingly rare, interest shifted to recreational exercise. Once again, the two pioneers, Professors Morris and Paffenbarger, were the first to look at this aspect of the subject.

Commencing in 1968, Professor Morris examined the effect of leisure-time exercise in a group of British civil servants. In articles published in 1973, 1980, 1987, and 1990, he has demonstrated that those who reported carrying out vigorous recreational activities in their leisure time, such as brisk walking (in excess of four miles or 6.5 kilometers per hour), swimming, badminton, jogging, digging in the garden, hill walking, and other similar activities at least twice weekly, had only one-third as much coronary disease as those whose recreational activities were more sedentary, and one-half the death rate from all causes. This benefit persists even when other risk factors, such as cigarette smoking, high blood pressure, diabetes, and obesity, are taken into account. Of course, the absence of these other

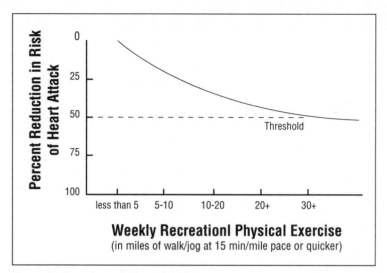

Figure 30: Exercise and Heart Attacks
The graph shows the percentage reduction of the incidence of heart attacks in Harvard University alumni according to their recreational exercise habits. The energy expended in various training activities is shown as miles of walking/jogging per week. (Source: Paffenbarger).

risk factors heightens the benefit of physical activity. For instance, exercisers who do not smoke have about one-fifth as many of heart attacks as sedentary subjects who are smokers. A history of engaging in vigorous athletics or team sports when young, which might indicate a genetic advantage, is not by itself associated with a lower incidence of coronary disease. "What matters," said Morris, "is the *current activity*, and compared with that the history when young is immaterial."

Professor Ralph Paffenbarger has been studying 58,000 Harvard college alumni since 1962. He reports that the incidence of death from cardiovascular and all causes in the most active men is 50% lower than in the least active (Figure 30). Evidence of protection begins to emerge once a total weekly energy expenditure of 500 kilocalories (about the equivalent of walking five miles [8 km] a week) is exceeded, and then increases with each additional 500 kilocalories until an expenditure of 2,000 kilocalories per week (20 miles [32 km] per week) is attained. Thereafter, little further benefit seems to accrue. From Professor Paffenbarger's data, the intensity of the walk (if we take walking as an example of leisure-time exercise) has to exceed 7.5 kilocalories a minute before the protective effect appears. For the sedentary middle-aged individual, this would mean walking at a pace of 15 minutes per mile (9.5 minutes per kilometer) or quicker. Obviously, other types of sports play or physical activity at the same intensity of effort would be just as effective, e.g., tennis, racquet ball, rowing, cycling, cross-country skiing, etc. Thus, there is considerable similarity between the findings of Professors Morris and Paffenbarger in terms of the intensity and amount of habitual physical activity required to protect one from coronary heart disease.

A 20-year follow-up carried out by Dr. Martha Slattery and co-workers from the University of Minnesota also studied the relation of leisure-time physical activity to coronary deaths and deaths from all causes in a group of 2,500 railway workers. The results showed that subjects who exercised regularly had a 20% lower death rate from CHD and from all causes compared with those who are sedentary. The amount of exercise required was equivalent to 20 miles of walking weekly. Another University of Minnesota researcher, Dr. Arthur Leon, followed 12,000 middle-aged men for 10 years and found that those who spent 45 minutes daily on light to moderate physical activity of any type were one-third less likely to die than their sedentary counterparts.

PHYSICAL ACTIVITY VERSUS PHYSICAL FITNESS

Although all these epidemiological studies have examined physical activity, none has measured the level of physical fitness that these activities confer. The shortage of such studies is understandable. An individual's physical habits can be ascertained from their occupation, a personal interview, and a questionnaire. Measurement of fitness, on the other hand, is a much lengthier procedure. It requires the use of equipment such as a stationary cycle or a treadmill, involves trained health professionals, and takes an hour or more of the subject's time.

Dr. Ruth Peters and her co-workers carried out fitness testing on 2,800 firefighters and law enforcement officers in Los Angeles County. They were divided into high and low fitness categories. Over a five-year follow-up period, the low fitness subjects had twice as many heart attacks as the high, even in the absence of other risk factors. When subjects who were unfit and possessed two or more of the major risk factors were compared to those who were fit and had the same combination of factors, the unfit subjects were found to have experienced six times the number of fatal and nonfatal heart attacks.

A collaborative study carried out between the universities of North Carolina and California determined the fitness level of 4,000 healthy men, aged 30 to 69 years, and divided them into four levels, or quartiles, the first quartile being the least fit and the fourth quartile the most fit. Over an eight-year follow-up, the death rate from all causes was much higher in those with the lowest level of fitness than it was in those with the highest (Figure 31). In fact, the first quartile compared with the fourth quartile had eight and a half times the death rate from all forms of cardiovascular disease, including strokes, and six and a half times the death rate from heart attacks alone. The results were found to be independent of smoking, cholesterol level, and blood pressure.

The men's fitness, or lack of it, corresponded to their reported level of exercise training and sports involvement, suggesting that a genetic resistance to heart disease

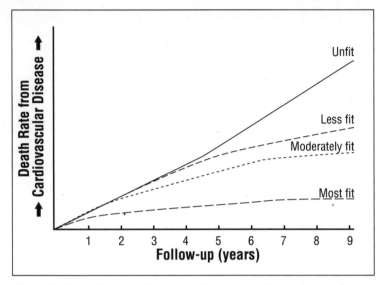

Figure 31: Death from Cardiovascular Disease According to Levels of Fitness
Over the period of observation, the least fit individuals showed the greatest mortality from heart attacks and strokes, while the most fit showed the lowest mortality. (Adapted from Ekelund *et al.*)

was not a factor. Also, if you look at the mortality curves in Figure 31 you will notice that they start to separate early and continue to separate even more over the course of the study, proving that the initial difference in fitness levels was not due to unrecognized heart disease at the beginning of the study. If it had been, then the greatest separation would have occurred within the first few years. Then as the sickest subjects died, the curves would have started to come together. A very similar study, which was carried out by Dr. Timo Lakka from the University of Kuopio in Finland, assessed the fitness level of 1,500 men aged 42 to 60 and then followed their course for four years. Over the period of observation, the most fit had one-third as many heart attacks as the least fit.

In 1989, Dr. Steven Blair and his colleagues from the Cooper Institute for Aerobics Research in Dallas reported on a study of 13,344 subjects (10,224 men and 3,120 women) who had been assessed and fitness-tested at the Institute. Over an eight-year follow-up period, the risk to the least fit men increased three times as much as the risk to the most fit, while the least fit women had more than a fourfold increase of risk compared with the most fit women. The greatest health gains occurred in those who progressed from being completely sedentary to the lowest level of fitness, with further but lesser gains as fitness improved. Fit persons with any combination of risk factors (cigarette smoking, elevated blood pressure, elevated blood cholesterol, diabetes, obesity, and parental history of coronary heart disease) had lower death rates than low-fit persons with none of these risk factors. The authors concluded " The results...support the hypothesis that a low level of physical fitness is an important risk factor for all-cause mortality in both men and women."

Physical fitness, then, has been shown to relate to physical activity. Furthermore, the fitter you are, the less likely you are to die from a heart attack. All very well, I can hear you say, but what if I have been sedentary for most of my life and decide to take up some form of physical activity in my late middle age? Can I get the same health benefits as someone who has exercised all their life?

Dr. Paffenbarger was the first to address this topic. In his early studies he showed that sedentary college students who adopted an active lifestyle reduced their risk of coronary disease to the same level as those who had always been active. He then looked at patterns of activity in men between 1962 and 1966 and again in 1977. They were then followed to 1990 to determine (1) whether they had changed their lifestyle and (2) their survival rate. The men who became active reduced their risk of dying from a heart attack by 50% compared with those who remained sedentary. This was constant across all age groups; the elderly, those aged between 65 and 84, would also seem to enjoy the benefit of becoming more active in their leisure time.

Dr. Blair investigated changes in fitness level of 10,000 men over an 18-year period, and found that for each minute improvement in treadmill test time there was a 10% reduction in mortality. Furthermore, while the benefit of quitting smoking was a 50% risk reduction, a favorable change in physical fitness resulted in a 60% reduction. Obviously, one would want to quit smoking and get fit. However, the message is clear, there is hope for all of us, even the most slothful of couch potatoes.

HOW MUCH EXERCISE?

Of course, as long as there is science, there will always be questions. We have now established that exercise has a myriad of benefits, and I have no doubt that in the coming years we will discover even more. The current discussion centers around how much exercise and how intense it should be. The traditional school of exercise physiologists have always maintained that in order to improve cardiovascular fitness one has to get one's heart rate up to a certain level, hold it there for 30 minutes or so, and repeat this three to five times weekly. The work of Professor Jeremy Morris tends to confirm this. He reported a reduction in the incidence of coronary heart disease mainly in those civil servants who indulged in "vigorous" (approximately 7.5 kilocalories per minute) leisure-time activities. Similarly, Professor Paffenbarger determined that the men who accumulated 2,000 kilocalories of physical activity weekly at a minimal intensity of at least 7.5 kilocalories per minute obtained the greatest benefit. If we take all the published work of both these experts, analyze their data, and express them in terms of a walking prescription for a middle-aged subject, we would be calling for a pace of 15 minutes per mile or greater for four miles (9.5 minutes per kilometer, for 6.6 kilometers), five times weekly.

On the other hand, Dr. Steven Blair has shown a graded decrease in coronary heart disease from the least to the highest level of fitness, the greatest reduction occurring from the unfit to the least fitness category. This implies that relatively low levels of physical activity can improve cardiovascular health. At the same time, however, Dr. Blair agrees that the more you exercise, the better the odds you will live longer. Finally, there is the view that health benefits accrue from the total amount of weekly or daily energy expenditure, irrespective of the intensity of effort. What can we make of all this? As yet, no one has all the answers. Any exercise is better than none at all, and up to a point, the more you do, the greater the return. The 1996 U.S. Surgeon General's Report "Physical Activity and Health" puts it like this:

"Recommendations from experts agree that for better health, physical activity should be performed regularly. The most recent recommendations advise people of all ages to include a minimum of 30 minutes of physical activity of moderate intensity (such as brisk walking) on most, if not all, days of the week. It is also acknowledged that for most people, greater health benefits can be obtained by engaging in physical activity of more vigorous intensity or of longer duration."

Finally, after nearly 50 years of epidemiological research, and thanks to the unceasing efforts of scientists such as Morris, Paffenbarger, Brunner, Blair and many others, the case for exercise in the primary prevention of coronary heart disease has been made. For the sake of completeness, and to be true to the scientific method, we must now ask ourselves the ultimate question. If fitness protects against heart disease, how does it work?

MECHANISMS BY WHICH EXERCISE TRAINING PROTECTS FROM CORONARY HEART DISEASE

Animal Studies

The hearts of wild animals are thicker-muscled and more copiously supplied with coronary blood vessels than those of their domesticated cousins (for example, wild ducks versus tame ducks or hares versus rabbits). By the same token, trained greyhounds and thoroughbred race horses have larger and more efficient hearts than the family dog or riding-school horse. Rats exposed to ten weeks of swimming training develop significant increases in size and number of their coronary arteries and branches. These changes are maintained so long as the rats continue to work out, but as soon as they stop training, the coronaries begin to return to their original state. Running training has been found to be just as effective as swimming.

Exercise can even increase the size and number of coronary arteries when one or more of the coronaries has been slightly narrowed. Dr. Richard Eckstein took a group of 90 dogs and, using surgical thread, artificially narrowed their coronary arteries to give them varying severities of nonfatal heart attacks. He then divided them into two groups, one group being confined to cages and the other put on an exercise program consisting of 20 minutes of running on a treadmill, five times weekly. At the end of a six- to eight-week period, he measured blood flow through the coronary arteries and noted that the exercised dogs had compensated for their narrowed blood vessels by developing new branches, known medically as collaterals. The sedentary dogs, on the other hand, showed no such effect. Eckstein concluded that "the judicious use of early and continued physical exercise may reduce the clinical manifestations of coronary disease."

The coronary anatomy of pigs is similar to that of humans. In one experiment, a group of pigs had a coronary artery narrowed so as to simulate coronary disease. One half were then trained, and the other half were not. Then the narrowed artery was closed off completely, mimicking a heart attack. In both groups, there was an immediate development of collateral vessels, but these were twice as plentiful in the trained as in the untrained animals. In addition, the area of damage to the heart muscle of the exercised pigs was only one-quarter the size of that in non-exercised animals.

Another approach has been to measure the effect of exercise training on the ability of heart muscle damaged from a heart attack to withstand the insult of recurrence. Dogs who were exposed to a "rehabilitation" exercise training program after a heart attack successfully survived a second one, whereas the non-rehabilitated dogs all died.

Much can be learned from the study of apes and monkeys, members of the primate family of mammals to which humans belong. Take the case of the longest-living gorilla in captivity, a resident of the Philadelphia Zoo. Since gorillas have the same life expectancy as humans, it was confidently predicted that he would live to sixty years or thereabouts. Actually, he died from a massive stroke at the age of 52. Even more disturbing, the autopsy showed that during his lifetime he had sustained a number of severe nonfatal heart attacks. Gorillas are vegetarians, and great care had been taken to provide him with the identical foodstuffs he would have enjoyed in the wild. This diet, totally free from saturated fat and cholesterol, should have protected him from coronary atherosclerosis. What had gone wrong? The answer lies in another aspect of the gorilla's lifestyle. In their natural habitat, gorillas cover large tracts of territory to forage for food. In captivity this was denied him, and it was the opinion of the zoo experts that the consequent lack of regular physical activity was the main factor contributing to his premature death from coronary heart disease. Does this mean that even the so-called ideal healthy heart diet cannot offset a life of sloth?

The work of Dr. Dieter Kramsch illustrates the other side of the coin. Over a period of four years, he fed a group of macaque monkeys a diet heavily loaded with saturated fat and cholesterol, the intent being to induce severe coronary artery disease. Half of the monkeys, however, were put on a training program consisting of one hour of running on a treadmill, three times a week. Over the four years of the study, a number of the non-exercising monkeys developed angina, as well as nonfatal and fatal heart attacks. By the end of the four years, all were found to have severe coronary artery disease. In sharp contrast, all the exercising monkeys remained in good health and at the end of the study were found, without exception, to have healthy coronary arteries, which were completely free of atherosclerosis and were, in many cases, larger in size than monkeys fed a normal diet. Not only that, but the exercisers had significantly higher blood levels of the "good" HDL-cholesterol and much lower levels of the "bad" LDL-cholesterol. What better illustration could there be of a good training program offering protection against a bad diet?

The Human Heart: Training Changes in Structure and Function

The human heart responds to exercise by changing in size and performance. It is nearly 100 years since the first observation was made that fit, long-distance skiers had large hearts, and the fitter and more successful the skier, the larger the heart. Subsequently, and with the increasing use of X-rays, most elite endurance athletes, such as long-distance runners, cyclists, and rowers, were also found to have cardiac enlargement. This finding led to the term "athlete's heart," meaning a heart that as a result of regular training was healthy, efficient, and powerful.

Unfortunately, in later years the term came to be synonymous with a diseased heart. How could this situation arise?

Until recently, physicians equated enlarged hearts with disease, because a failing heart will dilate, and thus increase in size. The heart of a hypertensive, which has worked for years against a high blood pressure, will develop enormously thickened muscular walls and will therefore also increase in size. Small wonder then that examining physicians, who were used to dealing with disease rather than health, were suspicious of athletes with big hearts, even though they could not find any evidence of the diseases that customarily cause the pathological enlargement.

Now that we have more sophisticated methods to observe the heart, we can better understand the exact nature of the enlargement that comes with training. Echocardiography (a form of X-ray using sound waves to picture the heart and its movements) has amply demonstrated that the ventricles of the endurance athlete's heart have a larger volume and capacity than is found in the sedentary subject. This has been particularly demonstrated in the case of long-distance runners and swimmers.

One of the most characteristic results of regular exercise is a drop in the resting and exercise heart rate. This lowering is referred to medically as *bradycardia* (Greek for slow heart). It is so characteristic of fitness that if it does not occur in the individual who is on a training program, you can be sure that the subject is either not adhering faithfully to the program, or that the training regime is badly designed.

To compensate for the lower pulse rate, the heart expels more blood per beat, or expressed physiologically, a greater volume of blood per stroke. This increase in stroke volume is another characteristic of the trained heart. The bottom line is a more efficient cardiac pump.

In animals, an increase in heart size is paralleled by a

proportionate increase in the diameter and number of branches of the coronary vessels, together with an increase in the capillary blood vessels that course through the substance of the heart muscle. In this way, blood supply keeps pace with demand. Does this also occur in humans? Clarence DeMar, a famous American long-distance running champion, died of cancer in his seventies; an autopsy of his heart revealed that his coronary arteries were unusually large. Although this may have been the result of natural endowment, it seems more likely that it was brought about by his many years of intensive training. Large coronary arteries are a distinct advantage in that they are unlikely to be blocked by even a lifetime's deposit of fatty atheromatous material.

It should also be noted that blood flows through the coronary arteries to supply the heart muscle *between* beats (that is, during diastole). Thus, the higher the heart rate, the shorter the period of diastole. Conversely, the slower the heart rate, the greater the proportion of time spent in diastole. Fitness bradycardia, therefore, is synonymous with a lengthening of diastole and thus an increase in coronary blood flow.

As if an improved blood supply to the heart were not enough, the fit exerciser has a further advantage over his or her sedentary counterpart. Fitness brings with it a reduction in the amount of blood the heart requires. Since the slowly beating heart muscle uses oxygen more sparingly, the blood flow does not need to be vigorous. It is a case of living well within one's cardiac budget.

The beneficial changes described above go a long way toward explaining why the fit heart is a healthy heart. But even if we do not possess the exotic equipment required to measure such changes, we would still be left with the simplest and yet one of the most important observations of all—the effect of training on the heart rate. We have already seen that training reduces the resting and exercising heart rate. It has a similar effect on blood pressure. We can obtain a very accurate index of the amount of work being done by the heart at any given time by multiplying the heart rate by the blood pressure. The result of this simple mathematical calculation is known as the Rate Pressure Product (RPP). Thus, if while sitting quietly reading this book, your heart rate were found to be 72 beats per minute, and your systolic blood pressure 120 mm Hg, then the work being carried out by your heart would be represented by an RPP of 8,640 (72 × 120 = 8,640). Assuming you were to put this book down, stand up, run vigorously on the spot for a few minutes so as to bring your heart rate up to 102 beats per minute and your blood pressure up to 140 mm Hg, then you would have increased your RPP, and therefore the amount of work your heart would be required to do, to a figure of 14,280 (102 × 140 = 14,280). Obviously, if training gives you a lower heart rate and a lower blood pressure for a given intensity of exercise, then you will have a lower RPP and the work load on your heart will be reduced. Physiologically, you would get more for your money. You will see later how this reduction in Rate Pressure Product for a given work load can have a powerful effect in relieving anginal symptoms in patients with coronary heart disease.

In addition to the benefit to the heart itself, fitness improves the cardiovascular system as a whole. The large muscles of the leg and trunk (the so-called skeletal muscles) develop a greater blood supply as a result of training. There is an increase in the size and function of the specialized cells (mitochondrial cells) that extract and utilize the oxygen from the blood. This improvement at the delivery end, as it were, of the oxygen transport chain means less effort is required at the source, that is, the pumping heart. The fact that these peripheral gains are possible and, indeed, inevitable in a good endurance training program explains why even individuals who have had very severe heart attacks can nevertheless benefit from a carefully prescribed training program.

THE EFFECT OF EXERCISE ON REDUCING CORONARY RISK FACTORS

Exercise and Cholesterol

In 1974, Dr. A. Lopez, Associate Professor of Medicine at the Louisiana State University Medical School, published a report describing the effects of a seven-week training program on 13 young medical students. There was a significant increase in HDL-C with training. Two years later, Dr. Peter Wood, an English biochemist working in the Stanford University School of Medicine, reported his investigation of 41 joggers who had been jogging in excess of 15 miles (24 kilometers) a week for a year. When compared with a group of sedentary men of similar age, all the joggers had considerably higher levels of HDL-C. He remarks in his article that "these very active men exhibited a plasma lipoprotein profile resembling that of younger women, rather than that of sedentary middle-aged men." Further reports verified Dr. Wood's findings.

In fact, not only the distance but the length of time the subject has been carrying out the exercise program may be important. A group of scientists from the University of Pittsburgh studied 35 active postal carriers who averaged approximately 25 miles (40 kilometers) of walking weekly over a duration of 15 to 28 years. Although keen exercisers would consider the pace to be almost leisurely, nevertheless the postal workers' HDL-C levels were significantly higher than average for the age-matched population.

Dr. John Duncan and co-workers from the Aerobics Institute carried out an interesting experiment on 100 premenopausal women. He divided them into four groups as follows: aerobic walkers (12 minutes per mile [7.3 minutes per km]), brisk walkers (15 minutes per mile [9.15 minutes per km]), strollers (20 minutes per mile [12.4 minutes per km]) and sedentary controls. The women walked three miles a day, five times weekly, for six months. At the end of the study, HDL-C measurements had increased to a similar extent in strollers, brisk walkers, and aerobic walkers. The investigators concluded that vigorous exercise was not necessary for women to obtain meaningful improvements in their HDL-C levels.

These studies, however, looked at healthy subjects. Can the same effect be achieved in patients suffering from coronary artery disease? The answer is decidedly affirmative. In 1979, Drs. Dan Streja and David Mymin of Manitoba, Canada, entered 32 middle-aged men suffering from coronary artery disease in a 13-week walk/jog program. Although there were no significant changes in total cholesterol, HDL-C levels increased significantly, and this "occurred in the absence of variations in diet, smoking habits, adiposity, or plasma triglyceride concentrations." Three years later, a report from the Cardiology Department of Victoria Infirmary, Glasgow, Scotland, described similar benefits in 19 post–heart attack men who were randomly allocated to an exercise program and were compared with 23 controls. The trial lasted for six months, and again the exercisers showed a significant increase in HDL-C levels. The level of exercise required was quite moderate, and in fact was a variation of the Canadian Air Force 5BX Plan.

I have also had the opportunity to study the effects of a one-year distance walk/jogging program on patients referred to the Toronto Centre, with similar beneficial results. Interestingly, our data demonstrated that the threshold dose of exercise needed to surpass the normal sedentary HDL-cholesterol values was 12 miles (20 kilometers) per week, very much as that found by other investigators. Furthermore, the pace, which ranged from 12 to 17 minutes per mile (7 to 10 minutes per kilometer), was less critical than the distance covered.

Dr. Zung Vu Tran from the University of Northern Colorado, has carried out a meta-analysis of 15 reports on the effects of exercise training on HDL-C levels in 490 heart attack patients. Their average age was 52 years, and they trained for an average of 24 weeks. Their HDL-C levels increased by 12%, a highly significant improvement. We know from other large cholesterol-lowering drug studies, such as the Helsinki Trial, that for every 1% increase in HDL-C, there is a 3% decrease in the risk of a heart attack. Thus, a 12% increase in these patients' HDL-C levels suggests that they have reduced the risk of a recurrent attack by 36%—a very gratifying benefit from the exercise training.

Exercise and Hypertension
Some years ago, a busy cardiologist who regularly refers patients to the Toronto Centre's program mentioned to me that he had taken up jogging 2 to 3 miles (3 to 5 kilometers), four times weekly. Apparently he had learned from a routine physical examination that he was suffering from mild hypertension. As he put it, "It was a case of taking medication or going on an exercise program, and as far as I am concerned, there was no contest." Approximately 20% to 40% of the population of the industrialized Western countries suffer from high blood pressure, and the overwhelming majority of these are classified as mild or borderline hypertensives (that is, they have a diastolic pressure between 90 mm Hg and 104 mm Hg and/or a systolic pressure between 140 mm Hg and 159 mm Hg; see Figure 13). My cardiologist friend, therefore, is in good company. Moreover, he also realized that all the antihypertensive drug trials showed that the benefit conferred to

mild hypertensives by drug therapy was marginal.

A number of the major exercise epidemiological studies have shown conclusively that the physically active are less likely to be hypertensive. Professor Paffenbarger's active Harvard alumni had a 35% lower risk of hypertension than their lazier counterparts. As if to vindicate the decision of my cardiologist friend, a 1989 study examined the incidence of essential hypertension in physicians who were members of the American Medical Joggers' Association and who jogged 10 miles (16 kilometers) or more per week and compared them with a group of non-exercising physicians. Both groups were carefully matched for age, gender, lifestyle, and socio-economic status. It turned out that only 7% of the jogging physicians suffered from hypertension, compared with 19% in the sedentary group.

Dr. James Hagberg has reviewed 47 studies that have assessed the effect of exercise training on subjects with hypertension. He found that 70% of the exercisers reduced their systolic blood pressure by an average of 10 mm Hg from an initial average pressure of 154 mm Hg. The average reduction in diastolic blood pressure was 9 mm Hg from an initial reading of 98 mm Hg. The effect of an exercise session was immediate, with the blood pressure remaining low for up to 12 hours after a workout. The more permanent effect was seen within weeks of starting the training regimen. The greatest benefit appeared to be in the 40-to-60 age group, with a suggestion that women obtained a greater benefit than men. Moderate-intensity exercise seemed to be as effective as vigorous effort. An ideal example for a middle-aged subject would be a two-mile brisk walk, five times weekly, or daily if possible.

Although the reductions in blood pressure as a result of exercise might appear modest, they are the same as those reported for weight loss, and greater than those for relaxation therapy, biofeedback techniques, and salt restriction. When used in conjunction with drug treatment, exercise can help reduce dosages. As a public health measure, it has the great advantage of being as cost-effective as you can get and, properly prescribed, safe from side effects. Table 1 (page 000) outlines the recommendations of the Joint National Committee on the Treatment of Hypertension with regard to lifestyle changes for the treatment and prevention of hypertension.

Exercise Training and Fibrinogen

We have seen that elevated fibrinogen levels are associated with an increased risk for coronary atherosclerosis and that stopping smoking can reduce fibrinogen levels. In fact, the beneficial effects of exercise on fibrinogen have now been extensively investigated. The Atherosclerosis Risk in Communities (ARIC) Study reported on levels of fibrinogen in 5,000 men and 6,000 women. Habitual physical activity was determined by interview and was graded from 1 (low activity) to 5 (high activity). There was an inverse relationship between level of activity and fibrinogen level, the lowest activity level having the highest fibrinogen measurement. This applied to both men and women. Furthermore, it was estimated that increasing physical activity by one unit would reduce the fibrinogen level by 0.3–0.4 grams per liter. A British study has calculated that a 0.1 gram per liter reduction in fibrinogen levels corresponds to a 15% drop in the risk of coronary heart disease. Thus, a decrease of 0.4 grams per liter could mean a 60% reduction in risk.

To date, at least five other large-scale cross-sectional (measurements were all taken once and at the same time) studies, five British and one German, have all found that the more sedentary you are, the more likely you are to have a high fibrinogen. And conversely, those who take regular physical exercise have low fibrinogen levels. Three longitudinal studies have looked at the effects of a training program on patients recovering from coronary artery bypass surgery, a heart attack, and individuals suffering from Type II diabetes. In the first, a 12% drop in fibrinogen levels was seen after six months of an aerobic training program which consisted of three 30-minute sessions a week. The maximum improvement was seen after just three months. Drops of 18% in fibrinogen after just one month of training were seen in a Japanese study dealing with 56 post–heart attack patients. The training program consisted of two 40-minute sessions of stationary cycling and walking daily for six days a week. Both these studies contained control groups who did not exercise, and who did not show any change in fibrinogen levels. The exercising Type II diabetes patients also obtained a significant decrease in fibrinogen after 14 weeks of aerobic-type training, but there was no control group in this study.

Exercise and Diabetes
Non-insulin-dependent diabetes (NIDD), also known as Type II diabetes, is a major risk factor for coronary disease. Diet and weight control are the cornerstones of treatment, but in recent years there has been more interest in the beneficial effects of exercise. Athletes and those who exercise regularly are known to be less likely to develop diabetes. Dr. Rose Frisch followed 5,400 college alumni into adult life and discovered that the prevalence of diabetes was 0.60% in the former athletes, compared with 1.3% for the non-athletes, despite the fact that the family history of diabetes was the same for both groups. One epidemiological study carried out in Fiji, where more than 20% of the population suffers from diabetes, showed that NIDD was twice as common in sedentary as in active men.

Dr. Bengt Saltin from the University of Copenhagen studied a group of men with glucose intolerance, a very early stage of Type II diabetes (see page 55). He found them to have a much lower fitness level than a group of age-matched normals. After completing three months of training, their fitness improved by 20%, and there was a distinct improvement in their glucose tolerance. After a further nine months of training, all members of the group had developed a perfectly normal glucose tolerance.

One of the most impressive examples of the value of exercise in NIDD is contained in a report from Dr. H.K. Takekoshi of Japan. A total of 103 NIDD patients were divided into three groups, one that did not exercise, one that walked leisurely for 30 minutes daily, and one that jogged for 30 minutes daily. All adhered to the same pre-scribed diet. They were followed for a period of ten years. At the end of that time, the jogging group showed no pro-gression of disease and was under very good control, with good control in the walkers, but only fair to poor control in the non-exercisers.

Exercise increases the body's sensitivity to insulin, which is why it is so important in the treatment of Type II diabetes (in which the patient becomes insensitive to their own insulin). Exercise also has a beneficial effect on Syndrome X (see page 57) by reducing obesity, high blood pressure, and high triglycerides, and increasing HDL-cholesterol. The antidiabetic effect of an exercise session only lasts for about 48 to 72 hours. On the other hand, the degree of benefit is unrelated to your level of fitness. In other words, the couch-potato Type II diabetic who goes for a brisk two-mile walk profits as much as the fitness advocate who goes for his fast two-mile run. There is some justice after all. In any event, all of this is taken into account by the American Diabetic Association's recommendation that Type II diabetes exercise at a moderate level, for between 15 and 60 minutes, at least three times weekly.

Exercise and Stress Control
Prolonged periods of stress—or distress, as I prefer to call it—can result in the sustained release of the "fight or

flight" stress hormones, adrenaline and noradrenaline. As we have seen, these substances increase the blood pressure, the heart rate, blood fat and blood sugar levels, and make the blood platelets sticky. A single bout of exercise puts these changes to the purpose for which they were intended—physical action. You can see how regular workouts repeated four or five times weekly can help us through the stresses and strains of everyday life. Certainly I find that if I hit a bad spot in the day and can go for a jog, everything begins to look a lot brighter, and what seemed to be an insurmountable problem gradually assumes more manageable proportions. Problems also have a way of solving themselves during a workout, largely because they are seen in perspective. When you are exercising, your mind is capable only of a superficial, holistic type of thinking; minutiae, trivia, and detail slip into the background, leaving you with only the prominent major points to consider. You no longer miss the forest for the trees.

Scientists have recently isolated from the brain and other nervous tissue a number of naturally occurring substances called peptides, which have opium-like qualities. One of these, beta-endorphin, has been reported to increase significantly in the blood after bouts of exercise. Furthermore, it has also been shown that regular training augments this response. Evidence at the moment suggests that the exhilaration, the feeling of relaxation, and the physical gratification felt as a result of a workout are due to release of these natural opiates.

Apart from these immediate benefits, however, there are the long-term effects of training on the catecholamine (adrenaline and noradrenaline) responses to stress. Work by Dr. Howard Hartley in the 1970s showed that after a physical training program the amount of noradrenaline released in response to physical stress was significantly decreased. A similar finding was reported by Professor Wildor Hollmann of Germany.

The Toronto Centre had an opportunity to investigate this benefit when we became involved in a multi-center randomized trial into the effects of an exercise rehabilitation program in post–heart attack survivors. The patients were randomized to control and exercise groups. Noradrenaline responses to various levels of work on the stationary cycle were measured on entry to the program and after one year. Exercise-induced noradrenaline levels were unchanged in the control group, but were significantly reduced, by 59% ($p = 0.05$), in the exercisers.

The value of such training-induced adaptations to stress cannot be overemphasized. Exaggerated surges of adrenalinelike substances have been blamed for the formation of intracoronary clots and for leading to heart attacks and cardiac arrest. If regular exercise can smooth out these surges, it may also protect against death from heart disease.

Exercise and Mood

Mood disorders are extremely common in our modern society. It is estimated that approximately 12% of the population of the United States suffers from depression, and about 4% from some form of anxiety neurosis. While psychotherapy, medication, and various relaxation techniques are frequently used as treatment, there is an increasing tendency also for physicians to prescribe a physical activity program. They know from practical experience that patients who exercise invariably "feel better." Is there any scientific evidence that there is a measurable improvement in mood?

There have been numerous published reports on the effects of an exercise program on depression. The early studies lacked scientific accuracy because of their poor design; they had no control group, exercise was inadequately monitored, and any beneficial effect of exercise they discovered was of dubious value. The later trials have been more sophisticated and their results more valid. A recent meta-analysis of 80 such trials by T. Christian North has established that regular exercise is a very effective antidepressant, superior in most cases to relaxation therapy, and often as effective as psychotherapy, and when combined with psychotherapy it enhances the improvement gained from psychotherapy alone. Aerobic activities such as walking, jogging, cycling, and swimming were found to be the most frequently prescribed and most effective forms of training. The antidepressant effect began after three or four months, and the longer the program lasted, the more pronounced the benefit. Finally, the trials that showed the largest decreases in depression with exercise were those dealing with coronary patients.

Exercise and Obesity
Although current weight reduction regimens inevitably stress calorie reduction through diet, they would be more successful if they emphasized energy expenditure as well. It was Dr. Jean Mayer, an authority on nutrition, who discovered that he could not make experimental animals obese by simply overfeeding them; they became fat only when he restricted their activity by putting them in cages. Of course, farmers have known this for generations. When they want to fatten their livestock, they don't merely increase their feed, they also limit their movement by enclosing them in small pens.

Obesity can be looked on as the result of an imbalance between energy intake and output. One would think that the more sedentary one is, the less one would want to eat. The opposite is the case. Studies have shown that sedentary employees eat more than moderately active workers. Individuals engaged in very heavy physical labor, such as lumberjacks, have greater appetites and consume more food than moderately active individuals, but they also burn more calories and so rarely become obese. Animal experiments have shown that rats that exercise for 20-, 40-, and up to 60-minute sessions at a time tend to eat less than their sedentary counterparts. Only when the exercise sessions exceed two hours at a time does their appetite increase. In summary, it appears that there is a level of activity below which our appetite does not relate to our energy requirements. Paradoxically, the less you do, the more you eat.

When we attempt to reduce body weight by diet alone, the weight loss consists not only of fat tissue, but also non-fat tissue (muscle and water). An exercise program, on the other hand, will burn fat, but by building muscle will increase non-fat body weight. For the first two to three months of training, the fat loss will often be balanced by an increasing amount of muscle and by water that is not being lost. Your bathroom scales may show little or no weight reduction, and if you don't take these physiological facts into account, you are likely to become very discouraged; you may even stop exercising altogether. During this stage, a better indication of your progress is the fit of your clothing.

Professor Michael Pollock of the University of Gainesville, Florida, advises that to lose weight, the workouts should last for at least 30 minutes, and the frequency should not be less than three to four times weekly. These guidelines have been confirmed by other experts in nutrition who have also found that walking, jogging, and cycling are among the most effective weight-reducing activities. The 30-minute minimum is probably due to the fact that after this length of time the muscles have switched over almost entirely from sugar to fat as their source of fuel. Swimming, for some as yet unexplained reason, does not reduce weight, although it is surmised that this may have something to do with the temperature of the water.

As a treatment for obesity, exercise has another distinct advantage over dieting alone. Exercise also improves a person's mood, whereas dieting alone often leads to an increased irritability and depression. The lifestyle change is also more permanent, and the weight loss more long-lasting.

To lose weight, most of us do best on a combined program of dietary restriction and exercise. Professors Zuti and Golding compared this combined approach to dieting alone and to exercise alone. The dieters reduced their intake by 500 calories a day. The exercisers increased their energy output by 500 calories per day, exercising five times weekly. The combined therapy group reduced their intake by 250 calories daily and increased their energy expenditure by 250 calories daily. At the end of 16 weeks, individuals in all three groups had each lost approximately 12% body weight. However, the composition of that loss was quite different. The two exercise groups lost more body fat and increased their lean body mass,

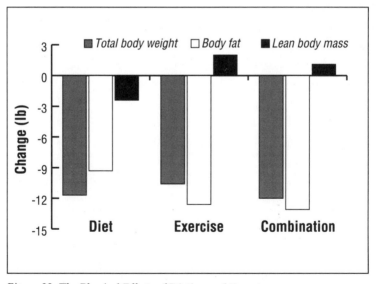

Figure 32: The Physical Effects of Dieting and Exercise
The graph shows the changes in body weight, body fat, and lean body weight brought about by dieting, regular exercise, and a combination of the two. (From W.B. Zuti and L.A. Golding)

whereas the diet group lost less fat and also lost lean body mass (Figure 32).

Exercise and the Endothelium

The role of endothelium (the layer that lines the coronary arteries) in coronary artery disease has assumed great importance in recent years. A healthy endothelium, by virtue of its ability to manufacture and release nitric oxide, can dilate the coronary artery so as to allow a greater blood flow and satisfy the demands of a fast-beating heart. It also acts as a barrier to the passage of LDL-cholesterol-laden scavenger cells, preventing them from burrowing into the wall of the artery and forming atherosclerotic plaques. Finally, it repels clot-forming platelet cells and prevents them from sticking to its surface. Indeed, we now know that the whole process of atherosclerosis commences with damage to the endothelial system, starting a chain of events that ultimately leads to a heart attack. Not only that, but a defective endothelium becomes a rogue endothelium; its response to an increased blood flow is not to dilate but rather to contract the coronary artery, narrowing its lumen and giving rise to the symptom of angina. Much of the benefit of stopping smoking, reducing high blood pressure, or lowering high LDL- cholesterol is due to the fact that these measures allow the endothelial cells to repair themselves and regain the ability to produce nitric oxide.

Obviously an active healthy endothelium is the first defense against coronary artery disease. It now appears that regular exercise may help the endothelium to maintain its healthy state. Animal studies have shown that exercise enhances the release of nitric oxide from the endothelium. Human studies as yet are few, since the whole topic is somewhat in its infancy. Nevertheless, a beneficial exercise-endothelial effect would explain, for instance, why an exercise session reduces blood pressure immediately, and more long-lasting reductions occur within a week or so of starting training. Increased nitric oxide production could dilate the blood vessels throughout the body, thus dropping the peripheral resistance and the blood pressure.

Alleviation of anginal symptoms is a well-known benefit of an exercise program, and was first described by the English physician William Heberden as long ago as the eighteenth century. Again, one explanation for this could be an exercise-induced enhancement of nitric oxide production. Patients suffering from heart failure are known to have a dysfunctional endothelium, with reduced capacity for the arteries throughout the body to dilate and a tendency for them to contract instead. A German study published in the American Heart Association's journal, *Circulation*, described how 12 chronic heart failure patients who underwent four weeks of training regained much of their capacity to dilate their blood vessels, due to an improved endothelial release of nitric oxide. Interestingly, six weeks after the training was stopped, the beneficial effect was lost, reminding us that an exercise program must be sustained if it is to be of any value.

These are exciting developments. It seems that every time we discover a new aspect of heart disease, exercise enters the picture. There is no doubt that we will hear a lot more about this subject in the future.

CONCLUSION

We now have conclusive evidence that lack of physical activity is a major risk factor for heart disease and that regular exercise can play a powerful protective role. In addition to improving the pumping power and efficiency of the heart, physical training has been shown to exert a favorable influence on the other coronary risk factors.

Improvement in fitness brings about beneficial changes in HDL-cholesterol and triglyceride levels, insulin sensitivity and glucose metabolism, blood-clotting mechanisms, stress hormone levels and endothelial function. Hypertension is improved and obesity reduced. The regular exerciser feels better and is more highly motivated to adopt a healthy lifestyle and abstain from smoking and a "junk-food," high-fat diet. Finally, this healthful prescription is free; your only investment is time. All in all, I think you will agree, an impressive list of benefits.

8. Exercise Training for Heart Fitness

So far we have talked about the cardiovascular benefits of physical fitness without defining what we mean by the term. A fit sprinter can cover 100 meters in under 10 seconds, but would probably have to drop out after the first mile of a 26-mile marathon race. Obviously, there are different types of fitness.

I chose the examples of the sprinter and the marathon runner not only because they are extremes, but also because they are perfect examples of the two categories into which muscle activity and physical fitness can be divided: anaerobic and aerobic.

Working muscles use only two fuels—carbohydrate (which is stored in the form of a substance called glycogen) and fat—both of which burn most efficiently in the presence of oxygen. So long as there is a steady supply of oxygen from the bloodstream, muscle action will continue until all the stored fuels are used. This type of muscle action, since it utilizes oxygen, is referred to as *aerobic*; literally, working with air.

The elite marathon runner who completes the 26-mile (42-kilometer) course in two to two and a half hours is an aerobic-type athlete. Initially, he runs on his stores of glycogen. However, since the body can only store about one pound (500 grams) of glycogen, he begins to deplete it after about 30 minutes of steady running. He then begins to draw on his fat stores. Incidentally, when almost all of the glycogen is gone the runner's legs will feel like lead; every step is an effort and he will need all his willpower to keep going—in runner's jargon he has, "hit the wall."

When a sprinter runs at top speed, his leg muscles use a process that burns glycogen *only* and does so in the *absence of oxygen*; this process is therefore referred to as *anaerobic*. Unfortunately, it can continue for no more than ten seconds, after which large quantities of a by-product called lactic acid build up in the muscle and slow down its contractions. Once the sprinter stops, the lactic acid has to be disposed of and the muscle fibers refreshed. This clean-up process requires oxygen. In other words, the oxygen debt built up during the ten-second sprint has to be paid back. Now you know why the sprinter, a carbohydrate-burning anaerobic athlete, can run the entire 100 meters without taking a breath, but once past the finish line doubles over, hands on knees, gasping for air and its content of oxygen.

Of course, most athletic activities require a combination of aerobic and anaerobic effort, in varying proportions. A 400-meter run will require an equal balance of both. A cross-country ski racer will perform aerobically on the flat, but anaerobically when climbing hills. For most of the 90 minutes of a soccer game, the level of activity is aerobic, interspersed with short bursts of speed requiring anaerobic muscle contusions. Nevertheless, we can say that long-distance running, cycling, and swimming are aerobic sports, depending largely on muscle endurance, whereas sprinting and weight-lifting are predominantly anaerobic sports.

From a medical viewpoint, the distinction is very

important because it is the aerobic activities, and the type of endurance fitness they confer, that lead to the cardiovascular benefits described in the previous chapter. Superior aerobic fitness is associated with an efficient oxygen transport system. The major links in this chain, you will recall, are (1) extraction of oxygen from the air by the lungs, where it becomes attached to the hemoglobin in the blood to form oxyhemoglobin; (2) in this form it is then pumped by the heart to the working muscles; (3) here it is transferred to a substance in the muscles called myoglobin, which shuttles it to the tiny "metabolic factories" in the muscle fibers called mitochondria, where (4) it is finally released in the form of oxygen again to fan the flame that burns the two muscle fuels, glycogen and fat.

PRESCRIPTION FOR AEROBIC FITNESS

If a physician were to offer you a medicine that was free, had no side effects, and was guaranteed to improve your heart, blood, and muscular system, would you accept it? I think you would. You might be surprised, however, to find that the medicine came neither in a bottle nor by injections, but was in fact a well-designed endurance-type exercise training program. If this sounds too simple, stop for a second and think of the incredibly complex changes exercise training can bring about. It can (i) increase the amount of hemoglobin in your blood; (ii) improve the efficiency and blood supply of the heart while at the same time making it more resistant to coronary heart disease; (iii) add to the network of blood vessels in the working muscles; and (iv) enhance the number and effectiveness of the muscle mitochondria so that they can burn fat more efficiently. All in all, you will agree, an imposing list of advantages.

When I prescribe a drug I specify its name, the strength

of the dose, the number of times it should be administered each day, and the duration of the treatment time. Writing a prescription for exercise is no different. I have to specify the mode or type of activity to be followed, the strength or intensity with which it must be performed, the frequency of workouts, and the duration of each workout.

Of these four components, exercise intensity is the most critical, since it determines the effectiveness and safety of the training program, a particularly important consideration for middle-aged people and those with heart disease. Let's consider it in some detail.

Intensity of Workout

If you want to train for an anaerobic event like a 100-meter sprint, you have to get your muscles accustomed to burning carbohydrate at a prodigious rate, without oxygen, for short periods at peak efficiency. Therefore, your workouts must simulate these conditions; they must be carried out at very high intensity and for brief bursts. The aerobic athlete, on the other hand, needs to conserve the body's meager stores of glycogen, start to burn fat (of which there is an almost unlimited supply) at an early stage of the training session, and ensure a constant supply of oxygen to the muscles. The workout should be carried out at an intensity low enough to permit it to reach the fat-burning phase, which occurs after about 30 minutes of exercise, without incurring an oxygen debt.

The intensity of the workout is thus determined by its duration. The higher the intensity, the sooner the exerciser has to quit. For instance, a novice exerciser may not be able to complete a 30-minute walk if the pace is a 15-minute-mile (9-minute-kilometer). On the other hand, that same exerciser may be able to stroll for 30 minutes at a snail's pace of, say, 60 minutes per mile (36 minutes per kilometer). However, such a low level of intensity would produce little or no aerobic training effect. Nevertheless, the concept that "duration determines intensity" is a useful one and is employed to advantage in the "out-and-back" training method. Here, the walker who wants to complete a 30-minute workout is required to proceed from a starting point, at a steady pace, for a period of 15 minutes, and then return by the same route at the same pace. If the starting point has not been reached by the 30-minute limit, then the outgoing pace was obviously too quick; if it is reached with time to spare, then the pace was too slow.

In the days before track coaches were exercise physiologists with postgraduate degrees from prestigious universities, you would often hear them exhorting their athletes to carry out a workout at "half effort," or "quarter effort" or "almost full effort." This instruction may have sounded vague to the uninitiated, but both the coach and the athlete knew what was meant. The principle was a good one and, in fact, is the basis for another approach we use today in aerobic training. The only difference is that we now measure and express effort in scientific units.

Oxygen Intake

Aerobic fitness is evaluated by measuring the maximum volume of oxygen the athlete can burn. This volume is expressed in liters of oxygen per minute, or if you take into account body weight, milliliters of oxygen per kilogram of body weight per minute (mL/kg/min). This maximum is referred to as the athlete's peak oxygen intake, or aerobic power; the higher it is, the better is the athlete's chance of competing successfully in an endurance-type event. Thus, an athlete with a maximum oxygen intake (often abbreviated to VO_2max) of 80 mL/kg/min will perform better in a long race than one with a VO_2max of 50 mL/kg/min. In other words, the former has a superior oxygen transport system. Once we have established someone's VO_2max, we can convert this into a running, cycling, or swimming speed, and then take one-half or one-third of this number to give the training pace equal to the old coach's one-half or one-third effort. For example, if you have a VO_2max of 35 mL/kg/min, then this tells us that you are capable of running a mile in 10 minutes or a kilometer in 6 minutes. A training pace that calls for two-thirds effort would be one which utilized 23 mL/kg/min ($35 \times \frac{2}{3} = 23$), which is equivalent to a 12-minute-mile (7.5-minute-kilometer) pace. The same calculation can be worked out for any percentage of VO_2max and expressed in the appropriate pace of any aerobic-type sport. To improve aerobic or endurance fitness, it has been established that the training workouts should be between 40% and 80% of one's VO_2max. At the lower end of the scale will be the very unfit, or the patient with coronary disease, while at the upper end is the fit athlete.

How do we measure maximum oxygen intake? The air around us contains 21% oxygen. Analysis of the air we expire, or breathe out, will show a reduction in this percentage; the difference represents the amount of oxygen consumed by our bodies. When you are relaxed or sleeping, this amounts to 3.5 mL/kg/min. Exercise physiologists often refer to this rate of oxygen utilization at rest as a MET*, and levels of activity above resting as multiples of a MET. For example, the oxygen cost of running a 10-minute mile (6-minute kilometer) is 35 mL/kg/min, or 10 METs (10×3.5 mL/kg/min). The more vigorously we exercise, the harder our muscles work, and the more oxygen they require. Ultimately, however, the point will be reached where the oxygen transport system can no longer cope with the muscles' increasing demands for oxygen. So far, and no further, they say. The most important limiting factor in this process—the link in the oxygen chain that determines when the body has reached its limit of oxygen utilization—is the heart. Once the heart has reached a point beyond which it cannot increase the amount of

*Metabolic Equivalent

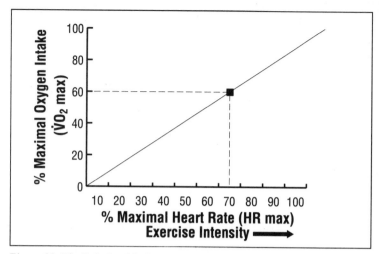

Figure 33: The Relationship Between Heart Rate and Oxygen Intake
Heart rate and oxygen intake increase together in a linear fashion as we exercise more and more vigorously. Because maximal heart rate is reached slightly earlier than maximal oxygen intake, the relative percentages of each value are slightly different. Here we see that 60% VO_2max equals 70% of HRmax.

blood it pumps per minute (maximum cardiac output), then greater physical effort is impossible. This is yet another expression of the fact that the level of your aerobic fitness is an index of your heart's health.

To test a person's maximum oxygen intake, we have to carry out an exercise test, which requires trained personnel and sophisticated equipment. We use a treadmill or a stationary cycle and increase the work stages every one or two minutes until the subject has to stop because of muscle fatigue. The level of oxygen intake at which this occurs is the subject's maximum oxygen intake, or aerobic power. Exercise testing, then, is the scientific way to determine aerobic power and is used to prescribe an effective and safe training program. Because of its complexity, however, the test is reserved for elite athletes or novice exercisers who are in the coronary-prone age group, or for those who actually have coronary heart disease.

Heart Rate

Simpler procedures involve the use of heart rates, which bear a predictable relationship to oxygen intake and therefore can be measured without the use of elaborate equipment. Since heart rate and oxygen intake increase at approximately the same rate in response to increments in effort, for most purposes we can use them more or less interchangeably. However, because the maximum heart rate is achieved slightly sooner than maximum oxygen intake, the percentages of maximum are not identical (Figure 33).

Everyone has a maximum heart rate that is related to his or her age. A 20-year-old's maximum heart rate is about 200 beats per minute, and a 70-year-old's about 150 beats per minute. A simple way to calculate your maximum heart rate is to use the equation 220 – (age in years) = maximum heart rate. This equation is not as accurate as that obtained by a maximum exercise test during which you actually achieve your maximum heart rate, and may be out by as much as 10%, but the method is accurate enough for general use in healthy individuals who are free from coronary heart disease. Using the percentage of maximum heart rate method, aerobic training intensity would range from 45% of HRmax for the unfit to 90% of HRmax for the athlete.

Yet another method of using heart rate to prescribe effort intensity is to take a percentage of the heart rate reserve (HRR), which is the difference between the resting and maximum heart rates. This percentage is then added to the resting heart rate to give the training rate. This method, called the Karvonen method, after its developer, has been shown to give a training heart rate which is much closer to that which occurs *at the same percentage of* VO_2max than would be obtained from simply taking a percentage of maximum heart rate. For example, to work out the HRR of 60% for a 48-year-old who has a resting heart rate of 72 by the Karvonen method: 220 – 48 (age) = 172 (maximum HR) – 72 (resting HR) = 100 × 60% = 60 + 72 (resting HR) = 132 HRR. You will note that this method gives a training rate higher than would be obtained by simply taking 60% of maximum heart rate (172 × 60% = 103). Resting heart rate is obtained by counting the pulse rate after sitting quietly for five minutes or so. It is customary to take two or three resting counts and then average them out.

Rating of Perceived Exertion

In the early days of the Toronto Centre's cardiac program, patients frequently reported that their doctors had cautioned them against activities that were too strenuous, or had told them that they could return to light work only. Such counsel, while well-meaning, was obviously too vague to be of much help. One of our tasks was to attempt to quantify work, not an easy task when you realize that what a lumberjack would consider to be light work would more than likely put his physician in hospital for a week.

In fact, it was situations such as this that led Dr. Gunnar Borg, professor of psychology in the University of Stockholm, Sweden, to devise a new way of looking at physical effort. Dr. Borg observed that injured lumberjacks who were judged on the basis of standard tests to be, say, 25% disabled often claimed that their disability was much worse than had been assessed. At first glance, one might suspect the workers of deception in order to gain additional industrial compensation benefits. However, in Borg's words, "Closer investigations seldom revealed any serious deception, but rather indicated that the patient was making a sincere effort to rate himself." This and similar observations in related fields led Borg to develop his Rating of Perceived Exertion (RPE) Scale, (Figure 34) in which the subject's perception of effort is rated numerically from 6, which represents almost no effort at all, through 20, the point at which further effort is impossible. The perception being asked for is one of overall exertion, rather than a feeling of effort or fatigue in any single part of the body. The numerical scale evolved from the fact that the original work was done with young men whose heart rates ranged from a resting of 60 beats per minute to a maximum of 200 beats per minute, and Borg discovered that the scale values of 6 to 20, when multiplied by 10, would approximate the heart rate of these individuals at the equivalent RPE. Since the scale is now used for a wide range of age groups, this simple pulse count is no longer valid. However, in any given individual, the scale does bear a remarkably consistent relationship to oxygen intake.

Original RPE Scale

6	
7	Very, very light
8	
9	Very light
10	
11	Fairly light
12	
13	Somewhat hard
14	
15	Hard
16	
17	Very hard
18	
19	Very, very hard
20	Maximal effort

Figure 34: Ratings of Perceived Exertion (RPE)
The original RPE scale. (From G.A. Borg)

Most people can be taught to recognize and reproduce this perception of exertion during their training workouts. The advantage of the method is that it allows for days when the conditions are adverse, such as high winds, hilly terrain, or excessive heat. On these occasions, the pace can be slowed to the required perceived exertion rating, and both the heart rate and oxygen intake will be maintained at the usual training level. The method may not be suitable, however, for all cardiac patients; it does not take into account irregularities in heart rhythm, or the effect of certain medications, such as beta-blockers, on perception of fatigue.

TYPES OF AEROBIC EXERCISE

Training for endurance fitness involves the repetitive movement of large muscle masses. Typical examples are brisk walking, jogging, swimming, long-distance cycling, and cross-country skiing. The possibilities are endless and depend on one's ingenuity and the climate in which one lives. The more complex the training activity, the more motor skill it requires, and the fewer people who will be able to undertake it. Also, since the ability to perform a particular sport varies widely, it is difficult to prescribe the effort intensity with true accuracy.

Walking and Jogging
I have used walking and jogging in the program at the Toronto Centre for 30 years, and have found these activities to be an ideal application for middle-aged subjects and for those with coronary heart disease. Walking and jogging give us greater returns of endurance fitness for a smaller investment of both time and money than any other activities I know. The skill required is minimal; the technique will be described later and can be learned in a matter of minutes. Special equipment is limited to a pair

of good shoes and, if you want to go first class, a sweat suit. You can walk and jog almost anywhere—through parks, along roads or sidewalks, or around neighborhood school tracks. In cold weather, you can use the local gymnasium, covered shopping malls, or even underground apartment garages (provided they are equipped with good fume-extractor fans). Opportunities are legion; the only basic requirement is motivation. I will deal with walking and jogging in greater detail in Chapter 12. Let us look now at other forms of aerobic exercise.

Outdoor Cycling

Cycling can be an excellent form of aerobic training. After all, some of the fittest aerobic athletes in the world are long-distance cycling champions. However, one needs good roads and, at least for cardiac patients, flat terrain to maintain a steady moderate intensity. In most large North American cities, cycle paths are a rarity, the motorists reign supreme, and one has to use extreme care. In cities with climates like Toronto's, the activity is limited to the summer months, since the roads in winter are frequently ice- or snow-covered.

If you are lucky enough to have access to attractive flat countryside, cycling may be the ideal exercise for you. Remember that the cycling speed has to be about twice that of running or jogging. For example, if your customary jogging speed is 12 minutes per mile (7.5 minutes per kilometer), you should be cycling at around 10 mph (16 kmph), or 6 minutes per mile (3.75 minutes per kilometer). An 8-minute-mile (5-minute-kilometer) runner would be required to cycle at 15 mph (24 kmph) to expend the same amount of energy.

Swimming

At first glance, swimming would seem to be the ideal aerobic training activity for the middle-aged subject, because it is non-weight-bearing and spares the knees, hips, and back. However, there are some drawbacks. Not everyone has access to a pool. Also, the energy expended depends on the proficiency of the swimmer. The beginner can squander more calories and use more oxygen thrashing from poolside to poolside than an experienced swimmer will use completing two smooth lengths. If heart rate is used to monitor effort intensity, it should be noted that the training rate should be 10 to 12 beats lower than used for upright exercise, and the distance should be only one-quarter of the dry land distance. For example, a 2-mile (3-kilometer) jogger whose training heart rate is 120 beats per minute would get an equivalent workout by swimming half a mile (about three-quarters of a kilometer) at a training heart rate of 110 beats per minute. The explanation for the lower training heart rate has to do with the body's horizontal position.

For patients with coronary heart disease, the temperature of the water is quite important. Most community pools are kept at 80°–84°F (26°–29°C). Cooler temperatures can cause angina or troublesome irregularities in heart rate. In older hypertensive patients, higher temperatures can be fatiguing and can sometimes cause fainting. Needless to say, high-risk patients who might be susceptible to cardiac arrest should be discouraged from using the pool.

Cross-Country Skiing

Long a popular sport in the Scandinavian countries, this activity uses both upper and lower limbs and produces highly fit aerobic athletes. One major study has also shown that regular practitioners live seven years longer than their sedentary counterparts. The intensity of effort required can be high, with a skier who covers the ground at 5 mph (8 kmph) using about as much energy as an 8-minute-mile (5-minute-kilometer) runner. Skiing, however, is highly seasonal, and the conditions can vary considerably, from ice through to loose or packed snow. Air temperatures may also be a problem for cardiac patients. Nevertheless, fun cross-country skiing is popular and becoming more and more a family event. Downhill skiing, incidentally, is not a totally aerobic activity and throws considerable isometric strain on the thigh muscles.

Stationary Cycling

The higher-priced exercycles are impressive pieces of machinery, full of "bells and whistles." Some monitor your heart rate, indicate when you are in the training range, simulate cycling up and down hills, advise you as to how many calories you have burned, etc. The only essential quality, however, is an easy and accurate calibration that will reproduce the desired pedal resistance, or work load, from workout to workout, day after day. It is this feature that separates a cycle ergometer (cycle work measurer) from just any stationary exercycle. Probably their greatest advantage is that they can be used indoors, leaving the exerciser with no excuse for not exercising during the extreme temperatures of winter and summer.

My experience using cycle ergometers for home exercise training programs, however, has been disappointing. I only know one individual, a highly motivated plastic surgeon, who has continued to use his exercycle regularly, five days a week, over many years. In general, most patients are enthusiastic for the first six months or so, but within a year the exercycle invariably finds its way from the study, to the bedroom, to the basement, where it eventually gathers dust for another year before it is sold to another enthusiastic neophyte exerciser. The first hint of its ultimate fate comes when the patient stations it in front of a television so as to watch a favorite program, or tries to set up some form of music-stand arrangement that allows a book to be read while cycling. Herein, of course, lies the crux of the problem. The exercycle is too convenient. The walker or jogger has to make time in the week to leave the home or office, and maybe change and shower. The day must be planned to include the workout, and this requires a change of lifestyle. The stationary cyclist *adds* the workout to the day's activities, whether to reading or to watching television. By doing so, the cyclist admits that exercising is an option, a luxury, and not something that has to take precedence over some other activity. Of course, if the cycling is carried out in a health club, then this situation does not apply. Not only is there the need to allow time for the visit, but there is also the companionship of fellow exercisers. "Spinning" is now a popular health club activity, in which groups of stationary cyclists intersperse steady-speed pedalling with bouts of high-intensity work, all to the direction and exhortation of the instructor. It is, of course, a form of interval training, first introduced 50 years ago by the Oxford University track and field coach, Franz Stampfl, who utilized it to prepare his protégé, Roger Bannister, for the first successful attempt on the four-minute mile. The basic principle is to train both the aerobic and anaerobic systems at the same time. The high-intensity short bursts of anaerobic activity make it unsuitable for the cardiac patient.

Solitary stationary cycling can be boring. There is no passing scene to gaze upon, no fresh air to breathe, no variation in terrain, no wind, no rain, no sun—no fun. So, if you choose this route for your exercise program, don't invest too much money at the start. If after a year or so you are still in the saddle, then treat yourself to a luxury model.

Motorized Treadmills
Treadmills have considerable attraction for those of us who live in extreme climates. The speed and grade can be

adjusted to replicate your customary level of effort, or in the more advanced models you can even program a combination of flat and hill walking or jogging. I find that after 45 minutes or so of treadmill work I am pretty bored, but you can't have everything.

There are certain key features we tell our patients to look out for in buying a treadmill. Make sure that the motor is powerful enough (1.5 HP) to maintain the speed of the belt at the required pace, irrespective of the user's body weight. The speed should have an adequate range, say 0.5 to 10 mph and the incline should adjust from 0% to a 16% grade. The change from one pace to the next should be smooth and gradual. The minimum "walking surface" or belt size should be 18" × 52" (45 × 130 cm). It should be two-ply or more, and cushioned for durability and comfort. Ideally, the deck should be pretreated, requiring little maintenance; others require lubrication on a regular basis to prevent sticking. Look for a high-grade steel frame and sturdy construction; if it looks flimsy—it probably is! Side rails should be placed so that they don't interfere with arm swing, and the display panel should be simple, easy to read, and convenient. An emergency stop button is essential. The price of treadmills has dropped considerably in recent years, although the addition of bells and whistles such as variable programming, heart rate monitors, calorie expenditure computers, etc., will rapidly add to the bill.

Don't hesitate to shop around. Specialty fitness stores will usually give you knowledgeable advice and help with the setup, whereas department stores may provide less expertise but a more competitive price. Try the equipment yourself and have the salesperson demonstrate all the features. Some stores may allow you to rent initially and apply the rental payments to purchase if you are satisfied and decide to buy.

Rowing Machines

These machines are becoming more popular. They are more expensive than a cycle ergometer and can provide a very strenuous workout. The semi-lying position adopted when rowing, as well as the heavy arm work required, puts more stress on the cardiovascular system than cycling. Heart rates and blood pressures are higher for a given oxygen intake. So, if you are a beginner, middle-aged, or have a history of cardiac disease, I would be cautious before investing.

Walking with Hand-held Weights

This activity, which has become popular in recent years, is intended to increase the oxygen intake, or intensity, of a walking prescription without having to increase the pace of the walk. Let us take an example. You have a VO_2max of 32 mL/kg/min. Your exercise training prescription calls for a workout intensity of 50% of your VO_2max, or 16 mL/kg/min, which works out to a walking pace of 4 mph (6.5 kmph), or 15 minutes per mile (9 minutes per kilometer). After you walk at this pace regularly for a while, your VO_2max improves to 40 mL/kg/min. To continue to train at 50% of your new VO_2max (i.e., 20 mL/kg/min), your pace will have to increase to 4.5 mph (7.2 kmph), or 13.5 minutes per mile (8.5 minutes per kilometer). However, this pace would require you to jog a portion of the workout, and it may be that for some reason, say a knee or a back problem, you cannot do this. Adding 3-pound (1- to 1.5-kilogram) weights to each hand will increase the oxygen cost of the 4 mph (6.5 kmph) walk by one MET, or 3.5 mL/kg/min, to 19.5 mL/kg/min, which is approximately the same as walking and jogging at a 13.5-minute-mile (8.5-minute-kilometer) pace. It should be noted, however, that merely carrying the weights will increase energy cost only slightly. You have to swing your arms, with elbows bent, and bring your hands up to shoulder height. For some, this parade-ground style feels unnatural and is embarrassing. It may also aggravate shoulder or elbow bursitis. More importantly, the arm work causes a disproportionate increase in blood pressure and heart rate, which may be a disadvantage for some cardiac patients. Weights heavier than 3 pounds (1.5 kilograms) will likely increase the chance of injury. I tend to prefer a natural walking or slow jogging action, but there is no doubt that for some the "heavy hands" approach has its place.

Rope Skipping

This activity was popular in the mid-1980s when it was proclaimed as one of the best ways to develop cardiovascular fitness. Since the skipping rope is easy to pack, and the activity requires little or no space, it seems ideal for business travelers and vacationers who want to keep up an exercise program while away from home. Unfortunately, for middle-aged adults who are unfit to start with, it has serious disadvantages. Apart from the fact that the technique takes some practice to perfect, it puts considerable strain on the legs, particularly the knees and calves. The most serious problem, however, is that it is impossible to carry out at a low intensity, which is where most of us want to start our fitness program. If you can't jog at a 10- to 12-minute-mile (6- to 7.5-minute-kilometer) pace, then you will not be able to skip for the 20 to 30 minutes required for aerobic training. In short, if you already have a good level of aerobic fitness and have learned the skipping technique, skipping is a good way to maintain your fitness while on the road. I do not advocate it for cardiac patients.

Aerobic Dancing, Dancercise

Popularized on television, video tape, and now part of every "Y" exercise menu, these continuous calisthenic activities are carried out to fast-tempo music and are usually very strenuous. Unless they are specially geared to the middle-aged, sedentary person, you should not participate unless you are very fit. The potential for leg injuries is also high, although the introduction of so-called low-impact aerobics has reduced this risk somewhat. The problem for the cardiac patient is that the intent of the activity is for the group to exercise in tempo; individualization can only be achieved by deliberately getting "out of sync" when the going gets tough. There is a natural tendency not to want to do this and so one is tempted to ignore symptoms.

Stair-Climbing Machines

These machines were introduced into fitness clubs in the 1980s. They are a modern version of stair stepping, except that they use two steps, which ascend and descend in response to the climbing action of the exerciser. The intensity of the workout can be modified by adjusting the speed of stepping and by changing the resistance required to depress the steps. Sophisticated versions include a computer program that varies the frequency and resistance of stepping to suit the weight and fitness of the subject, gives the number of miles climbed, number of calories burned, etc. Other models also include bars for hand gripping. The concept here is good, in that the intention is to use all the muscles of the upper and lower limbs for a good aerobic training effect. Note, however, that the strain on the thigh muscles can often be greater than that imposed by stationary cycling.

Buying a stair-climber can be more arduous than purchasing a stationary cycle or a treadmill. Stair-climbers have different types of drive mechanisms, including belts, cables, and chains. They can be manually or electronically run. The manual models use either hydraulic oil-filled shocks or air-filled shocks (the former are more durable).

All in all it might be a good idea to try a climber in a gym for a while before deciding on whether or not to buy.

Step Aerobics

Step aerobics is frequently a feature of health club fitness classes. They say there is nothing new under the sun, and certainly this latest vogue in exercise equipment is an example of this adage. Bench stepping has been used to measure cardiovascular fitness since the 1920s. The current products on the market generally consist of a bench, about 4 feet (1 meter) long and 1 foot (30 centimeters) wide, which can be adjusted for height from about 6 up to 12 inches (15 to 30 centimeters). The exerciser steps up and down to a count of four. Intensity of effort can be adapted to suit the individual by regulating both step height and rate of stepping. It has been calculated that at 80 steps per minute the subject is using the same amount of oxygen as if jogging at a 10-minute-mile (6-minute-kilometer) pace. A cadence of 120 steps per minute equals an 8.5-minute-mile (5-minute-kilometer) pace. Advocates of this system maintain that there is less impact than jogging, although when I tried it myself I found it hard on the knees (an age-related problem, no doubt). By pumping the arms and adding weights, you can increase the intensity further.

DURATION AND FREQUENCY

There are two other components to be considered when prescribing a training program: the length of the training session, and the number of times it should be carried out per week. As we have seen, the duration of the workout should be at least 30 minutes, with a goal of 45- or even 60-minute sessions. More intense levels of activity may achieve the same training effect with shorter sessions, but the sedentary, middle-aged individual, or the patient with coronary heart disease, is better advised to make haste slowly. There is also the matter of weight reduction. Glycogen stores begin to drop after about 10 minutes of exercise. By 30 minutes, glycogen provides no more than half the energy required, and from then on the body begins to draw more and more on its fat stores. Have you ever seen an obese long-distance runner? You probably never will. The training sessions are so long that all excess fat is burned, with the result that long-distance runners have the lowest percentage body fat of all athletes. It is duration rather than intensity that burns calories. The name of the game, then, is long slow distance, or LSD.

As for the frequency of training, four to five times a week seems ideal. Nowadays, competitive athletes train seven days a week, and sometimes twice a day. Such excessive measures may well pay off when only yards or meters and seconds separate the world's best and the third-rater, but the added 1% to 2% improvement that seven-days-a-week training gives hardly makes it worth the effort for the average person. On the other hand, individuals who train less than twice a week make minimal progress. I realize that the Surgeon General's Report calls for 30 minutes of moderate exercise on most, if not all days of the week. However, once we progress to 45 or 60 minutes of vigorous exercise, two rest days will be a welcome respite.

RESISTANCE TRAINING

While aerobic training is the major component of all cardiac rehabilitation programs, there is an increasing tendency to add weight training to the exercise regimen. This is particularly valuable for those who require upper- or lower-limb muscle power, either on the job or for recreational activities such as racquet sports or skiing. It used to be thought that all forms of weight training were dangerous for the individual with coronary disease. We now know that this isn't so, and that many patients can benefit from a medically prescribed weight program that is tailored to the individual.

When prescribing a resistance training program we need to specify the mode (free weights or weight-lifting machines), the intensity (the amount of the weight and the number of times it is lifted), and the frequency (or number of workouts weekly). Most cardiac rehabilitation programs use free weights in the form of dumb-bells, which are hand-held, or barbells, which are held with both hands. Multistation weight machines have some advantages, but they can be quite expensive. As for frequency of training sessions, two to three times weekly is customary.

As with aerobic training, intensity plays a major role, and to understand how it works in resistance training we need to explain a few simple technicalities.

The maximum number of times a weight can be lifted before the onset of fatigue prevents further lifts is known as a repetition maximum, or RM. Obviously, the RM will depend on the weight being used. A weight that can be lifted once only is referred to as 1-RM, one that can be lifted five times as 5-RM, and so on. Intensities of 3- to 6-RM favor the building of muscle strength, whereas lightening the load and increasing the number of repetitions to 12- to 20-RM makes for increased muscle endurance and stamina.

The American Heart Association recommends about eight resistance exercises that train the major muscle groups of the body; i.e., arms, shoulders, chest, abdominals, back, trunk, hips, and legs. Each exercise should consist initially of one set of 10 repetitions, increasing gradually to 15 repetitions (10- to 15-RM). Once 15 repetitions can be accomplished easily, the weight can be increased by an additional 5%. Workouts should be carried out two to three days a week.

Since the establishment of 1-RM requires considerable effort on the part of the patient, many cardiac rehabilitation programs avoid this by starting with a weight that will allow 10 repetitions comfortably; this is roughly equivalent to about 40% – 50% of 1-RM.

Having said all that, it is very important to note the following:

1. Cardiac patients should enter into a weight-training program only after medical clearance, and then only under the direction of trained professional personnel.
2. The use of ECG and blood pressure monitoring is generally indicated, at least during the initial sessions.
3. Heart attack and heart surgery patients should wait at least six weeks before beginning weight training, and they should have a level of aerobic fitness that permits them to walk a mile in 16 to 17 minutes comfortably.
4. Patients with the following conditions should not weight train:
   • severe heart failure
   • uncontrolled and symptom-related extrasystoles
   • severe disease of the heart valves
   • moderate to severe hypertension (systolic ≥ 160 mm Hg, or diastolic ≥ 100 mm Hg)

While more research needs to be carried out on the benefits of weight training as an adjunct to aerobic type training in cardiac rehabilitation, we do know that it can enhance muscle strength and endurance, improve exercise capacity, and boost psychological well-being. There is also some evidence that it might help to increase insulin sensitivity. However, it has only minimal, if any, effect on peak oxygen intake, and there is no evidence that it improves the coronary risk profile by increasing HDL-cholesterol, reducing triglycerides, dropping high blood pressure, lowering stress hormones, or reducing fibrinogen levels.

9. The Cardiac Rehabilitation Program

"There is no way you can go back to your old job," said the physician.

Bill H., a 39-year-old construction worker, stared across the desk in disbelief. "What can I do?" he said. "I don't know any other trade. How will I get by?"

Firmly, the doctor reminded him of the facts. Bill had just been discharged from hospital after his second serious heart attack. The first was a year ago. Bill's father had died at the age of 42 from a heart attack. One older brother had died, also in his forties, from a heart attack, and another brother had sustained a heart attack at age 38.

It was essential, said the doctor, that Bill take all sensible precautions to see that he had recovered completely before returning to heavy physical labor. His wife would have to go out to work, and he would have to stay at home to look after their two children, prepare their meals, and carry out the routine housework. This approach was hard for Bill to take, yet his common sense told him that his doctor was right; he was not in shape to withstand the physical strain of his job.

As the months went by, Bill became more and more morose. Never what you would call an abstainer, he began to drink heavily. Instead of benefiting from the enforced rest from work, his health became worse. He began to notice chest pains, some of which he thought were angina and others he thought were nerves. He was irritable with the children and downright unpleasant to his wife. Fortunately, his doctor was astute enough to realize that things weren't working out the way he had hoped. The doctor still felt that return to work was not the answer; neither was sitting at home all day.

"The less I do, the flabbier I get," said Bill, plaintively. "At this rate, I'll never work again."

Doctor and patient gazed speculatively at one another, each trying to find a solution.

Then Bill had a thought. "Why not send me to one of the Y's fitness classes? Wouldn't that build up my strength again?" As he spoke, his voice became more enthusiastic. Already he was seeing himself active and vigorous again, participating in the games and sports he had enjoyed at school.

The physician was torn. There was no doubt a fitness program would boost Bill's morale, but what of the safety factor? How could he entrust Bill and his damaged heart to a fitness class geared to the needs of essentially healthy individuals? Then, a thought stirred in his mind. Hadn't he read somewhere recently that a local rehabilitation center had just started a postcoronary rehabilitation program? He promised Bill he would enquire further and let him know the outcome the next day.

The doctor was true to his word, and the following week, Bill was waiting in the lobby of the Toronto Centre. It was 1968, and he was one of the first patients referred to the new exercise rehabilitation program for heart attack patients.

Ken S. was 54 years old. He had "had it with doctors." And his doctors had almost "had it" with him. A highly successful executive, Ken was a prime example of the uncooperative patient. He had just been discharged from hospital after recovery from his second heart attack. The first was only three months earlier, and his reaction at that time had been truly macho—hang tough and stay in there fighting. In Ken's terms, this meant denying that he was suffering from anything other than a minor setback. He discharged himself from hospital earlier than his cardiologist advised and returned to work the following week. Shortly after this, he put himself on an exercise training program as outlined in a popular book on fitness.

Since he considered himself a rather fit individual, he skipped through the precautionary chapters of the book, and started halfway up the training table at a level suitable for those whose fitness rating was good.

In short, Ken did all the wrong things. Small wonder that six weeks later, while on a business trip and shortly after attempting a 9-minute-mile (5-minute-kilometer) run through Stanley Park in Vancouver, he experienced severe chest pain. On his return to Toronto, he was diagnosed as having sustained another, and this time more extensive, heart attack. He was lucky enough to survive, and one would have thought that after that experience he would have adopted a more cautious approach. Obviously, caution was not in his nature; if nothing else, one had to give him an A for persistence. He was still determined to work, worry, and play at his customary pre-attack level.

He presented his hapless cardiologist with an ultimatum: "Tell me how to get fit and strong again, or send me to someone who can."

His physician, feeling that Ken had had a great deal more luck than he deserved and anxious to protect him from further excesses, recalled reading of an exercise rehabilitation program being carried on in the city. He recommended the program to Ken.

"My God," said Ken. "Rehabilitation! You mean basket weaving?"

"Not quite," said his doctor.

The rehabilitation program to which these men were referred was unique in that it stressed prolonged endurance exercise. If Ken expected basket weaving, he was in for a shock. From the outset each participant would be asked to walk for half an hour, at a pace based on performance on an initial exercise test, five times a week. Within a matter of weeks, the time would be increased to one hour. The ultimate goal would be four miles (6.5 kilometers), five times weekly.

The starting level and rate of progression would depend upon the results of rigorous cardiorespiratory fitness testing. The exercise plan would be carefully tailored to accommodate each person's twofold need: developing endurance fitness, and doing so with minimal risk to an already damaged heart. The individual would be given a prescription specifying duration, intensity, and frequency of exercise.

All patients would be expected to attend exercise classes regularly until they achieved their fitness potential. During these supervised sessions, they would be observed by physicians, therapists, and physical educators to see how they performed. If they developed cardiac symptoms, they would be examined again or their electrocardiogram would be monitored while they exercised. They were all instructed in the art of taking their own pulse, reading a stopwatch, pacing themselves, and jogging in an easy and relaxed manner so as to avoid minor injuries to muscles, tendons, and joints.

Physician-led discussions would deal not only with the physiological and medical aspects of endurance training, but also the significance of exercise-induced symptoms associated with coronary heart disease. Individual advice on whether to participate in other sports such as squash, weight lifting, tennis, or curling would be available. Lectures and discussions would center on such risk factors for coronary heart disease as cigarette smoking, blood cholesterol, and high blood pressure.

Bill, Ken, and the others were going to discover that many of the sports in which they had taken part, under the impression that they were good for their health, were actually of little value in attaining true worthwhile fitness; and that a set of singles tennis played on odd occasions through the year to a perspiring, gasping, knee-trembling finish did more harm than good. But more importantly, they were going to find that they were expected to work constantly and assiduously on their own, changing their lifestyle to accommodate five sessions of exercise every week. Their reward? Something that money cannot buy. They would experience the sheer physical elation of being fit.

The Origins of the Program
In 1768 the English physician, William Heberden, stirred up the medical world when he presented a scientific paper entitled "Some Account of a Disorder of the Breast" at a meeting of the Royal College of Physicians. In it he described, for the first time, one of the presenting symptoms of coronary heart disease. He called the symptom angina pectoris, Latin for "spasm of the chest," pointing out that it was brought on by physical exertion, particularly after a meal, became worse if the activity was continued, but was relieved by standing still. Heberden maintained that angina was symptomatic of a serious condition that carried a grave prognosis. To this day the paper has been praised for its simplicity, as well as its observational and descriptive accuracy. Bear in mind that this paper was written before there was any real understanding of the role played by the coronary arteries in heart disease. Nevertheless, it marks the historical starting point for our look at cardiac rehabilitation.

Heberden lived to the age of 91, and during his practicing life, he encountered one hundred cases of angina pectoris. Keen observer that he was, he carefully documented the following item about one of his cases. "I have little or nothing to advance.... for the treatment of angina but did know of one patient who set himself the task of sawing wood for half an hour every day and was nearly cured." He had recognized what appeared to be a paradox. How could a symptom which was brought on by exercise be cured by exercise? Of course, he had no answer for this, but he was probably the first to describe the benefit of exercise training in coronary heart disease.

There the matter rested until 1854, when William Stokes, Professor of Medicine at Trinity College in Dublin, described his "pedestrian cure" for heart disease in his classic medical textbook, *Diseases of the Heart and Aorta*. It consisted of slow walking on level ground, the pace to be prescribed by the physician, with undue breathlessness and chest discomfort to be avoided. As the patient's condition improved, the duration and speed of the walk was increased. Stokes reported considerable success with this method, describing how some of his patients progressed to the stage where they could easily manage brisk walking over hilly terrain. His teaching was largely forgotten until the latter part of the nineteenth century, when it was taken up again by Dr. Oertel of Munich, who combined the walking therapy with a weight-reducing diet for his heart patients.

By this time, however, a totally different philosophy to illness had evolved, and it was to bury the exercise approach for the next hundred years. In 1863 the London surgeon Dr. John Hilton published a book called *Rest and Pain*. In it he maintained that the most effective way to help a patient recover from an illness or a surgical procedure was to allow the body full scope to use its own natural defense mechanisms. This could be achieved only, he said, by enforcing strict bed rest. Unfortunately, his admonition was carried to the extreme. Patients recovering from heart attacks were kept in hospital for as long as eight weeks and bore the full brunt of this form of treatment. Immobilization was the order of the day; little, if any, movement was permitted—except the mandatory daily bowel movement. Even this was performed between the sheets, with the patient perching precariously on the ubiquitous bedpan (an endeavor, ironically, later found to be more energy consuming than using the toilet).

One of the first to take issue with the strict bed rest philosophy was Dr. William Dock, a California physician who during the 1940s published an article entitled "The Evil Sequelae of Complete Bed Rest." In it he stated bluntly that lying flat for days on end could lead to severe depression, pneumonia, blood clots in the leg veins or lungs, back problems, muscle wasting, softening of the bones, and even sudden cardiac death in heart attack patients who were struggling to use a bedpan.

In 1954, two Harvard Medical School cardiologists, Dr. Samuel Levine and Dr. Bernard Lown, described their revolutionary "armchair" treatment. Of 73 patients admitted to hospital for a heart attack, 15 were taken out of bed and nursed in an armchair on the first day, 30 on the second, 18 on the third, and the remaining 10 on the fourth to the ninth days after their attacks. Contrary to the prevailing fears of the time, they did not suffer ruptured hearts and premature death. In fact, they all made excellent recoveries. One of the most spectacular features of the treatment was their patients' enhanced sense of well-being and relief from anxiety. The period of convalescence was shortened considerably, and there was an earlier return to work. This experiment marked the turning point in the treatment of heart attacks and led to the widespread acceptance of early mobilization during the 1960s. Mind you, patients were still kept in hospital for up to four weeks or more, and the mobilization was, by today's standards, quite timid. For example, one paper described a regimen which called for a 15-minute slow walk, twice daily, but not commencing until *four weeks* after the heart attack, while another describes the nurse putting the patient's limbs through a series of *passive* exercises *two weeks* after the attack.

Nevertheless, it was a start. By the 1960s, pioneers such as Dr. Herman Hellerstein of Cleveland, Dr. John Naughton, then of the University of Oklahoma and now Dean of Medicine at the University of Buffalo, New York, and Dr. Peter Rechnitzer of the University of Western Ontario, Canada, were reporting successful results with postcoronary patients entered into walking and calisthenic programs. Further afield, Dr. Brunner of Israel compared a group of 64 patients in his exercise program with another group of 65 postcoronary patients who had not followed any exercise regime. Over the period of a year, there were four recurrences and two deaths in the exercise group; the non-active group had nine recurrences and seven fatalities. Dr. Victor Gottheiner, also from Israel, published a most comprehensive report of his experience in exercising 1,100 patients with coronary heart disease. Using a variety of endurance activities such as brisk walking, jogging, cycling, swimming, and rowing, he was able to demonstrate that his methods were both safe and effective.

The Toronto Program
How did the program at the Toronto Centre get started? The remarkable escalation in the incidence of heart attacks, together with the realization that the survivors were still in peril from a fatal recurrence, led me in 1967 to realize that something more than routine follow-up by a physician was required. If all the risk factors were to be covered, a change in lifestyle was required. Granted, such risk factors as high blood pressure, diabetes, and high

blood levels of cholesterol can be controlled by regular visits to the physician, but matters such as physical activity,
diet, stress, giving up smoking, and making a major
lifestyle change require more prolonged attention, help,
and advice.

The Toronto program was introduced in 1968; the main
component would be exercise, around which would be
built educational aspects and various behavioral inter-
ventions designed to encourage a healthy lifestyle.

The type of exercise chosen was walking, progressing
where appropriate to jogging. For patients who had difficulty walking, we used stationary cycling and swimming.
In recent years, we have also added strength training with
light weights for patients who need to improve their
upper body strength or those who suffer from extreme
muscle weakness. Walking and jogging still remain our
favorite forms of aerobic training. They require little in the
way of equipment or expensive facilities; their intensity,
duration, and frequency can be controlled, and they are
excellent builders of endurance fitness.

Postcoronary exercise programs are plagued by poor
attendance and high drop-out rates. After the first flush of
enthusiasm, the exerciser finds that regular attendance
disrupts his or her social or business commitments. This
problem is worse in a large city, where one often has to
travel long distances on traffic-clogged roads and highways. The answer was to reduce the number of weekly
medically supervised sessions to the minimum and have
patients work out on their own the rest of the week. After
all, if one cannot be taught to exercise prudently when
away from the watchful eye of the physician, how can one
be expected to cope with the inevitable sudden physical
stresses and strains of normal everyday living? Also, if safe
exercise rehabilitation programs are to become universally available, the logistics of the situation make it
mandatory that medical staff be used for the maximum

good of the maximum number; physicians, nurses, and therapists are in short supply, and their services should be deployed carefully.

We decided, therefore, that patients would exercise as a group at the Centre under medical supervision only once a week. Since a greater frequency of training is needed for attainment of endurance fitness, four additional home workouts would also be required. This approach has worked very well. Our patients have become fit and attend the weekly session with great regularity; indeed, the program has one of the lowest dropout rates recorded.

All patients must be referred by a physician. The referral documents, together with hospital reports and electrocardiograms, are carefully studied by the Centre's doctors to see if there are any reasons not to exercise. The patient is then brought to the Centre for a complete examination. His or her height, weight, muscle power, and percent body fat are recorded, together with a routine electrocardiogram. Finally, the patient performs a maximal exercise test, either on the cycle ergometer or on the treadmill. A walking/jogging exercise plan is prescribed on the basis of the test results. The prescription states the specific distance to be covered and the time it should take. It calls for five workouts a week, one of which is carried out under supervision.

All patients are required to keep an exercise log that they hand in regularly. This log records their current prescription, the distance and time of each workout, and their pre- and postworkout heart rates. It also has space for noting any adverse symptoms experienced during a particular workout. The logs are read carefully by the treatment staff, and the distances, times, and heart rates are carefully charted for each patient. In this way, progress can be easily gauged at a glance. Adverse symptoms are underlined in red and immediately passed through to the physician for his or her attention. If necessary, the physician will phone the patient to clarify some remark or even to suggest that exercise pace be reduced, or exercise training be stopped, until the next supervised session.

Traditionally, isometric training has been excluded from the cardiac patient's program, for what are good physiological reasons. A static muscle contraction that involves 75% or more of maximum effort shuts off the blood supply to that muscle and results in a compensatory increase in heart rate and blood pressure. This could be potentially harmful to the ischemic heart. However, in recent years, there has been increasing interest in strength training. We now know that cardiac patients may undertake *supervised* and *prescribed* weight-training programs without risk, provided that the weights are relatively low in respect to maximal effort (usually no more than 50% of full effort), and that they are capable of being lifted ten times in succession without excessive strain. Care should also be taken to avoid breath-holding during weight lifting since it can lead to an abrupt rise in blood pressure and put an extra strain on the heart. A good indication for weight-training is in preparation for return to an occupation that involves considerable arm work, or where the individual wants to take part in throwing or racquet sports.

Our studies have shown that the patient often experiences a great improvement in mood and morale within weeks of starting the program. Nevertheless, a period of at least six months is required for full physiological benefits to appear. When they have reached a satisfactory level, patients are "promoted" to a group that attends the Centre only once every fourth week.

Due to the steady demand from out-of-town physicians for cardiac rehabilitation, we have also instituted an Outreach Program. The patient travels to the Centre for testing, is instructed in the performance of the exercise prescription, and reports his or her progress by means of mailed-in exercise logs. Progressively heavier training workouts are prescribed as the patient gets fitter, returning for retesting after three, six, and twelve months.

A Home Program

Over the years, the two most common questions asked of me by patients who do not have access to a supervised exercise program or a cardiac rehabilitation facility are: what is a safe starting level of exercise, and how does one safely increase this to improve the training effect? Obviously, there is no single answer to either question. The starting level will vary with the individual, depending upon initial state of fitness, the severity of the heart attack, age, and the presence or absence of symptoms. Any increase in the training prescription will depend upon training response, expressed subjectively in feelings of well-being, and objectively in heart rate response to the workout and to repeated stress tests. However, over the years, we have learned to streamline our exercise-prescribing technique and have developed a series of tables especially designed for heart patients. These are contained in this book, which is the final extension of the program. It is an attempt to reach individuals who are coronary-prone, or who have coronary heart disease and want to start an exercise program but lack expert guidance. Obviously no book will substitute for personal supervision and contact, but I hope this one will help you avoid at least some of the more dangerous pitfalls. The tables, together with a set of progressing nomograms, should provide safe and effective guidelines for the intelligent lay person. Used with the accompanying remarks on training techniques, they constitute a home version of the Centre's program.

Women in the Program

The number of women referred to the Toronto program

has steadily increased over the years. Nevertheless, women still constitute only about 20% of our current patient caseload. Mind you, that number is not inconsiderable, particularly when you recognize that we now admit a total of 1,700 cardiac patients to the program annually. Nevertheless, when you realize that about as many women as men suffer heart attacks, the referral rate should be much higher. One reason for this relatively poor referral rate might be that attendance at the rehabilitation classes could be more of an inconvenience for the housewife or a working woman with household responsibilities—or, probably more likely, an inconvenience for her spouse! It is also possible that the woman herself, or her medical adviser, or both, feel that rehabilitation is unnecessary, or is unlikely to be of help.

Nothing could be further from the truth. Actually, the woman who has had a heart attack or undergone coronary artery bypass graft surgery is often more incapacitated from angina, depression, anxiety, and poor physical conditioning than her male counterpart. If she had a job before her illness or surgery, she is less likely to go back to it. As a housewife, she often still has difficulty with physical tasks around the home. In our experience, women derive the same benefit as men from rehabilitation. For example, we have compared the before and after body measurements and fitness levels in 272 women and an equal number of age-matched men, all recovering from a heart attack or bypass surgery, who attended the Toronto Centre. Compliance to the program was excellent, and the same in both groups; the women attended 71.3% of all sessions, the men achieved 71.1%. In terms of body measurements, the women did better than the men, losing a greater percentage of body fat and gaining more muscle bulk than the men. Fitness levels, as determined by exercise testing, increased by 15.5% in the women, and by 17.4% in the men, a highly statistically significant gain for both groups. This, then, is hard objective evidence that women can adhere to a program, and make just as much progress as men.

WHAT TYPES OF PATIENTS SHOULD BE REFERRED FOR EXERCISE REHABILITATION?

Now let's look at what particular groups can benefit from cardiac exercise rehabilitation.

After a Heart Attack

Historically, cardiac rehabilitation has been aimed at people who have had a heart attack, and these patients still constitute 36% of all referrals to our program. However, with the advent of techniques to improve blood supply to the heart muscle, such as bypass surgery and angioplasty, additional groups of patients have been added.

Many post–heart attack patients make uncomplicated recoveries and do not require additional procedures. They are referred to a rehabilitation program because they or their physicians recognize the need. Some require help to return to heavy labor or to vigorous recreational activity. In others, restoration of self-confidence is needed to attain full recovery. I believe that all low-risk patients should at least be assessed for rehabilitation, and preferably by the rehabilitation team. Coronary atherosclerosis is a progressive disease, and my experience is that most will benefit from a program of risk factor reduction and physical conditioning. Even patients who consider themselves fit may be exercising at an inappropriately high intensity and will benefit from a more structured program.

After a Bypass

As bypass surgery has become more common, so the number of such cases referred to the program has increased, until at the time of writing they constitute 33%

of the total. Surely there can be no better expression of the way in which exercise rehabilitation has been accepted as being complementary to medical and surgical treatment of heart disease.

I have always believed that for a person to gain the full benefits of coronary artery bypass graft surgery, the patient should receive advice after surgery on exercise and lifestyle change. Unless the risk factors associated with the presence of the disease in the first place are effectively removed, then it is not surprising that some patients develop symptoms again. In our experience, the patient who adheres to the precepts of the rehabilitation program has a better long-term surgical result. Other programs similar to ours have had the same experience. Indeed, one group of Japanese investigators found that exercise prior to surgery and continued for three months afterwards significantly improved the chances of the graft remaining open.

After Angioplasty

Patients who undergo angioplasty are likely to underestimate the chronic nature of their disease. They see the procedure as a quick fix and fail to recognize the necessity for rehabilitation. Many of the benefits obtained from rehabilitation by CABG patients are also applicable to those who have undergone angioplasty. In general, an angioplasty patient can commence exercise rehabilitation a week after the procedure. Until recently the insertion of a stent was accompanied by the administration of the potent anti-clotting agent warfarin (Coumadin) and this was continued for three months. This deferred referral to an exercise rehabilitation program. However, the anti-platelet agents aspirin and ticlopidine (Ticlid) have replaced Coumadin and thus patients with stents are accepted for training as soon after surgery as those without stents.

Heart Transplantation Patients

One of the leading centers in the world for heart transplant surgery is Harefield Hospital in London, England. The surgeon, Sir Magdi Yacoub, is a firm advocate of postsurgical exercise rehabilitation, and in 1984, at his invitation, we initiated a joint research project between Harefield and the Toronto Centre. This program involved the exercise testing and training of English transplant patients by senior members of the Centre's staff. Every three months, we spent two weeks in Harefield working with the new patients and reassessing previous ones. In the intervals between these visits, communication was maintained by mailed exercise logs, in a manner similar to the system adopted for patients on the Toronto Outreach Program. The results were excellent and were published in the official journal of the American Heart Association, *Circulation*, in 1988.

Disease of the Heart Valves

Apart from congenital defects, the commonest cause of valve disease is rheumatic fever, a condition which largely affects the young but which is now rare in the western world. However, it is still a problem in African and Asian countries, and so can still be seen in immigrants to North America from these regions. Nowadays, as the population ages, we are seeing more valve disease as a result of wear-and-tear degenerative changes. Whatever the cause, the diseased valve gives rise to problems either because the flaps become stiff, and so restrict blood flow (stenosis) or they fail to meet, allowing blood to leak backwards (regurgitation). By and large the heart can compensate for the altered hemodynamics, but over time flow problems may become more severe, the heart begins to fail, and corrective surgery may be indicated. After the valve is repaired, or replaced, and normal heart function restored, then all is well. However, some patients may have experienced considerable physical limitations as a result of their valve disease, and even though their surgery has been successful, they remain in a deconditioned state. These individuals make ideal candidates for exercise rehabilitation.

Chronic Heart Failure
For many years it has been an established practice for patients who have suffered from *heart failure* or who have poorly functioning ventricles to avoid all exercise. However, in recent years the situation has been reevaluated. Once out of the acute stage of failure, and if there is no leg swelling or evidence of backup of fluid in the lungs, then a medically prescribed, carefully supervised exercise program has been shown to alleviate symptoms, improve exercise capacity, and increase feeling of well-being and morale. In 1996 we reported in the British specialty journal, *Heart*, our experience in training a group of such patients over a one-year period. They all did extremely well, showing significant improvement both in fitness and in quality of life as early as 12 to 16 weeks into the program. There were no adverse incidents. Experience is still limited, however, and research is continuing in a number of centers around the world. In the meantime, it would appear that a combination of the new heart failure drugs and a prudent exercise training program can greatly improve these patients' outlook.

SAFETY OF EXERCISE REHABILITATION

Recognizing that patients with coronary heart disease, both those with or those without symptoms, are more likely to suffer a fatal heart attack or a cardiac arrest than their healthy counterparts, it is reassuring to know that the safety record of medically supervised cardiac exercise programs such as ours is excellent.

We have adopted a number of routine precautionary measures at the Toronto Centre in order to minimize the risk of an accident. The supervising staff is not only efficient and observant, but works hard to create an informal and friendly atmosphere during exercise sessions so as to avoid feelings of tension or anxiety. The patients are also advised to adhere to the following exercise rules:

- always warm up and cool down;
- avoid extremes of heat and cold;
- train regularly without excessive peaks of activity;
- avoid intensive competition;
- adhere to the prescribed limits;
- reduce the exercise load when symptoms such as angina or frequent skipped beats occur, or during times when anxiety or tension is present; and
- report all symptoms, and particularly episodes of light-headedness or blackouts, no matter how brief.

WHO SHOULD NOT EXERCISE?

The vast majority of coronary heart disease patients, whether they have had a heart attack or suffer from angina, will benefit from a medically prescribed sensible exercise program. So also will the middle-aged individual who has any of the coronary risk factors (and that means most of us over the age of 40), or who has a family history of heart disease. There are, however, some people who should absolutely not exercise, either for cardiac or non-cardiac reasons. There are others who need to take extreme care. Exercise is possible for them, but it must be modified and carried out under supervision.

Cardiac Contraindications to Exercise

As I have said, these are few, and your physician should be your final guide.

1. A *recent heart attack.* Since the myocardial infarction scar takes about four to six weeks to become firm, *vigorous* activity prior to that time may cause a thinning of the scarred wall. If this occurs, the wall will become weak and bulge outwards every time the healthy muscle wall surrounding it contracts inwards. This bulge is known as an aneurysm. If the aneurysm is small, it is of little consequence. However, if the aneurysm is large, it can weaken the pumping power of the heart, a condition that may be associated with dangerous irregularities of heartbeat. A large aneurysm can also prevent safe participation in a good exercise training program in the future. In some cases, a large aneurysm can be cured surgically by cutting out the thinned scarred area.

   This is not to say that normal activities of daily living, including comfortable walking, should not be permitted before the six-week period, but entry into a supervised training program should not take place until after an exercise test.

2. There is no role for exercise in *acute heart failure.* In this condition, the heart is unable to pump the blood around the body efficiently; the symptoms are extreme breathlessness and swelling, or oedema, of the legs. Heart failure is not a common complication of coronary artery disease, but when it does occur, it is usually in association with a very severe heart attack resulting in extensive damage to the heart muscle. Even then, healing of the infarct may result in complete recovery in pump efficiency, at which time exercise again becomes permissible. In recent years, patients who have suffered from attacks of heart failure and have been stabilized by some of the newer medications are

undertaking carefully monitored exercise rehabilitation programs with very good results. However, more research is needed in this area, and until we have accumulated additional information, these patients should not be encouraged to exercise on their own. Their place is in a specialized center under the guidance of skilled exercise specialists.

3. As we have seen, a *large aneurysm* of the heart wall is a bar to exercise. Aneurysms may also occur in the walls of the large blood vessels (for example, the aorta), and their presence here also precludes vigorous training. There are, of course, cases in which small aneurysmal bulges are present; here the question of whether or not to exercise becomes a matter of fine judgment. Again, such individuals should not attempt to regulate their own program, and skilled supervision by a physician is essential.

4. Patients who develop *rapidly progressing anginal pain* should not exercise. Any change for the worse in the *pattern* and *incidence* of exertional pain may well be the warning of another heart attack. A typical example might be a patient who finds that angina is induced at a much lower level of exertion than usual. Or, alternatively, a patient who generally suffers from exertional angina only, but then finds that he or she is being awakened during the night with chest pain. To exercise under these circumstances may well be to invite disaster.

5. The heart muscle can sometimes be involved in *generalized infections*, giving rise to a condition known as myocarditis, or inflammation of the myocardium (the medical ending "itis" means "inflammation of"). This infection can occur in acute rheumatic fever, or in viral infections such as infectious mononucleosis (glandular fever) or even influenza. Since exercise is never advised during acute infections, it is obviously even

more dangerous when the infection involves the heart. While your physician will be the one to diagnose myocarditis and will certainly ensure that your physical activity is limited until the condition has cleared, it should be stressed that mild subclinical myocarditis may be common in association with a number of viral-type infections. For this reason, I insist that all individuals on an exercise program stop training whenever they develop any influenza-like illness, particularly one that is accompanied by muscle pain, tenderness, and a rapid heart rate. Exercise should never be performed in the presence of a fever, and to be on the safe side, the temperature should have returned to normal for 72 hours before working out again.

6. *Markedly irregular heart action* that is aggravated by exertion is a deterrent to training, especially if the electrocardiogram shows that these ectopic beats are emanating from more than one area in the heart. These "multifocal" ectopics, which are aggravated by strenuous exertion, can on occasion lead to fatal ventricular fibrillation, and exercise should not be undertaken until the condition has been controlled by suitable medication. Compensation can be made for lesser degrees of rhythm irregularity by modifying the training regimen.

   It should be stressed that there can also be benign irregularities in the heartbeat. These are often present from youth. The distinction can only be made accurately if they are seen on an electrocardiogram, but a rough rule of thumb to their identification is that these irregularities are often present at rest but disappear as the heart rate increases with exercise.

7. In certain types of *valvular heart disease*, especially those that lead to severe narrowing in the region of the aortic valve, exercise training may not be advisable. Coronary heart disease does not affect the valves in

this manner; rheumatic fever in childhood is the usual offender. Occasionally, both valvular disease and coronary artery disease can co-exist, in which case one has to be guided by the severity of the valvular difficulty.

8. Patients suffering from recent cases of *blood clots* occurring either in the lungs (pulmonary embolism), or in the peripheral arteries or veins (thrombophlebitis), should not be exercising. Physical activity may bring about further clots, or extension of the existing ones.

9. *Repeated bouts of heart failure* may, in the long run, give rise to a dilated enlarged heart. This will show up on the X-ray and also on an echocardiogram. Where the enlargement is pronounced, there will be no benefit from training. The stretched heart muscle has no reserve left and so is incapable of benefiting from even measured small doses of exercise stress.

10. Exercise therapy is of little value in the condition of *complete heart block*. Here, the electrical conduction system between the upper and lower chambers of the heart is nonfunctioning, with the result that the atria and the ventricles beat independently. Furthermore, an increase in heart rate does not occur when the subject exercises. In such a condition, a pacemaker, or artificial rhythm conductor, is inserted. This brings the heart rate up to a set level and may also, depending on the type and design, permit it to accelerate in response to exercise. Those individuals who have been fitted with an appropriate pacemaker can benefit from an exercise program.

11. Most patients with high blood pressure do well on an exercise program. However, if the *hypertension* is very marked, *in excess of 200/110 mm Hg,* and cannot be controlled by medication, then vigorous exercise *could be* harmful because it drives the pressure up higher and may cause a stroke.

12. Certain forms of *congenital heart disease,* especially

those that are associated with a bluish discoloration of the face, feet, and hands (cyanosis), are contraindicators to exercise.

Noncardiac Contraindications to Exercise

1. If you suffer from *severe uncontrolled diabetes*, you should avoid exercising until your condition is stabilized. A blood glucose level of 16 mmol/L (300 mg/dL) is a contraindication to exercising, or a blood glucose of 13 mmol/L (240 mg/dL) if ketones are present in the urine.

2. Some individuals suffering from *epilepsy* may find that exercise, by bringing the body to a state of "arousal," may increase the frequency of seizures. In such cases, the problem may be solved by altering the dosage or type of antiseizure medication, or by modifying the intensity or duration of the training session. Often a satisfactory modification can be achieved by a process of trial and error.

3. Sustained exercise makes increased demands on the lungs, kidneys, and liver, and in *diseases* where the functions of these organs are severely compromised, exercise is obviously contraindicated.

4. The acute stages of various types of *arthritis*, such as rheumatoid arthritis or gout, are treated by appropriate medication and rest. During these acute phases, exercise will do more harm than good. However, during the quiescent phase, suitably modified exercise programs will be beneficial.

    The more crippling type of osteoarthritis may be aggravated by weight-bearing activities such as running or jogging; in these situations cycling or swimming may be more appropriate. In passing, however, I should note that long-distance runners have been shown to have a lower incidence of osteoarthritis in their hip joints than the population at large; this is due to the fact that movement keeps the protective cartilaginous lining of the joint surfaces healthy and well nourished. Our legs were meant for walking—not sitting.

5. *Chronic low back trouble* can be exacerbated by jogging or by certain types of calisthenics. However, factors that are even more aggravating are obesity, running on an uneven surface, wearing unsuitable running shoes, or performing activities that involve twisting movements of the spine: the golf drive, the tennis serve, squash, or badminton. If a careful watch is kept for flare-ups, and activity is slowed with the advent of suspicious symptoms, back strength should develop to the stage where a full program of walking/jogging can be sustained without problems.

6. There are a number of other conditions in which exercise may be ill-advised. These include various rare neurological, muscular, and glandular diseases. In any event, the physician must be the final judge in these matters, and his or her advice and permission are essential for any patient with coronary heart disease who wishes to embark upon the training system outlined in this book.

10. The Benefits of Exercise in Cardiac Rehabilitation

We have already dealt with exercise training as a way of reducing or eliminating many of the risk factors for coronary disease. We have also seen that the training reduces resting and exercise heart rates, increases the amount of blood the heart can eject with each beat, reduces resting and exercising blood pressure, enhances the efficiency with which the muscles can extract oxygen, and increases maximal oxygen intake. We will now look at the extent to which these changes apply to the cardiac rehabilitation patient.

Psychological

It is not uncommon for someone who has survived a heart attack to experience bouts of depression. This is a perfectly natural response, and usually cures itself in a matter of months. However, it has been my experience that an exercise training program can speed up the recovery process. In fact, one of our exercise studies published in the *Canadian Medical Journal* demonstrated this accelerated recovery, not only in the mildly depressed, but also in a group of more profoundly affected patients. Since then, we have shown similar benefits in heart transplantation recipients and, more recently, patients with chronic heart failure.

Apart from the psychological boost one gets from being able to look on the bright side of things again, it now appears that there is even more at stake. Dr. Nancy Frasure-Smith, consultant psychologist with the famed Montreal Heart Institute, has conducted a number of landmark studies into the effects of post–heart attack depression on prognosis. She found that depression could be a harbinger of future problems—more specifically, another heart attack. If her further research proves this to be so, then the ability of postcoronary exercise rehabilitation to alleviate depression could well explain at least some of its proven capacity to reduce the incidence of a fatal recurrence by some 25%.

Heart Performance

Since the heart is a major link in the oxygen transport chain, it is not surprising that patients admitted to the program after a heart attack frequently have a low maximal oxygen intake on the initial exercise test. Over the course of the program, they show an average increase in VO_2max of 25%. A higher VO_2max means more than just an improved performance in a laboratory test; it means an increased capacity to lead a full, active life.

RELIEF OF ANGINA

We mentioned earlier that William Heberden, an eighteenth-century English physician, was the first to record the fact that regular physical activity could relieve the symptom of angina. One of his angina patients put himself on a training program of wood-cutting for half an hour every day, "and was very nearly cured." Obviously the fact that angina, a symptom brought on by exercise, could also be cured by exercise, struck Heberden as being something of a paradox, odd enough to warrant drawing to the attention of his fellow physicians.

Angina is the result of an imbalance between the flow of blood through a narrowed coronary artery and the demands of the heart muscle for blood. It occurs when the heart has to increase the pace and force of its contractions, generally in response to a bout of physical exertion, or sometimes as the result of an emotional event which gets our adrenaline flowing.

If we want to cure angina we can, at least theoretically, approach the problem in two ways. We can either *reduce the demand* imposed by the heart on the narrowed coronaries, or we can *increase the blood supply* to the heart through the coronaries. Immediate short-term relief of angina can be provided by the use of nitroglycerine, which *temporarily* dilates the coronary arteries, thereby increasing the supply, while at the same time dilating the arteries and veins throughout the body, dropping the pressure against which the heart has to work, and thus reducing the demand. Beta-blocker medication on the other hand, which drops heart rate and blood pressure at all levels of effort, also prevents angina, but only by decreasing the heart's demand for blood. One of the most consistently reported benefits of exercise training in patients is the eventual relief of exertional angina. Does training work by reducing demand, increasing supply, or both?

Reduction in Demand—Rate Pressure Product (RPP)
Exertional angina generally occurs at a particular Rate Pressure Product (heart rate × systolic blood pressure). The RPP at which angina appears is referred to as the patient's *anginal threshold*. Because training reduces the heart rate and blood pressure, eventually the patient can reproduce that same level of work without reaching the

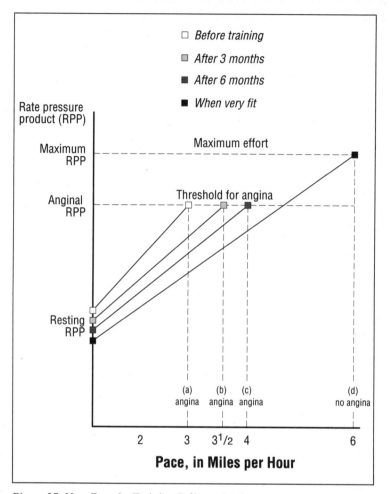

Figure 35: How Exercise Training Relieves Angina
This patient reaches the Rate Pressure Product (heart rate X blood pressure), which produces angina at a walking pace of three miles per hour (A). After three months of training, the resting and exercising RPP drops, and the anginal threshold is not reached until a pace of three and a half miles per hour is attained (B). After six months, four miles per hour is attained before the onset of angina (C). Here, angina is being relieved by a reduction in cardiac work (RPP) at a given level of effort, i.e., a reduction in *demand*. Sometimes a patient becomes so fit that he can exercise to an RPP which is greater than the anginal threshold, yet experience no symptoms (D), circumstantial evidence that there has been an increase in *supply*, i.e., coronary blood flow has improved.

RPP anginal threshold. The heart's demand for blood has been reduced.

Take the example of a patient who gets anginal pain when walking a mile (1.6 kilometers) in, say, 20 minutes, at which pace the heart rate increases to 110 beats per minute, and the systolic blood pressure to 130 mm Hg, giving an RPP of 14,300 (110 × 130). Let us say that after training for two months, the 20-minute walk can now be accomplished at a heart rate of 102 beats per minute and a systolic blood pressure of 126 mm Hg. The RPP is now 12,852, well below the anginal threshold (Figure 35). Ultimately, as fitness increases and the RPP drops even further at all submaximal work rates, the patient is able to carry out all the normal activities of daily life, including vigorous activities, without ever reaching the anginal threshold.

Increase in Supply
There is another mechanism by which training could reduce the symptoms of angina. You will recall that blood flows through the coronary arteries during the period of diastole, the relaxation phase between heartbeats. A trained slow-beating heart has longer periods of diastole, thus allowing more time for coronary blood flow to occur. This additional circulation time is often sufficient to compensate for the reduction in flow caused by atherosclerotic narrowing. In a sense, this is a way of increasing supply.

Collateralization
From time to time, coronary patients become so fit that when we exercise-test them, they achieve a heart rate and blood pressure (Rate Pressure Product) higher than their previous anginal threshold and yet do not develop angina. This indicates that, despite the increase in demand, the supply remains adequate. Therefore, the ability of the coronary circulation to provide the heart

with blood must have improved. There are two ways this could happen. Either there has been growth of new coronary artery branches that detour the blood flow around the narrowed segment (like a natural bypass), or the narrowing itself has opened up as a result of shrinkage in the size of the atheromatous deposit. The first process is referred to as *collateralization*, and the second as *regression*.

Coronary collaterals are tiny blood vessels, no thicker than a fine hair, which vary in length from a few millimeters to about 3 centimeters. Under normal circumstances, they carry little or no blood. However, if the coronaries start to become narrowed as a result of atherosclerosis, the collaterals respond by gradually growing in size and number so as to compensate for any reduction in coronary blood flow. The greater the growth in collaterals (collateralization), the less likely is the coronary narrowing to cause angina, or to lead to a heart attack if the narrowing closes off altogether. Animal studies have shown that regular exercise training is a powerful stimulus to collateralization. As the animal becomes fitter, the collaterals increase in size and number (by the same token, when training stops, the collateral vessels gradually shrink). Even when the animal is entered into an exercise training program *after the coronary arteries have been artificially narrowed*, extensive collateralization is often seen, and this has been shown to improve survival after an experimentally induced heart attack.

The evidence for training-induced collateralization in humans has been less easy to obtain, mainly because the size and location of the collateral vessels make them difficult to see on a coronary angiogram. However, the technique of thallium exercise testing can provide circumstantial evidence for collateral growth in coronary patients entered into an exercise rehabilitation program. Briefly, the patient with angina has an exercise thallium test at the start of the rehabilitation program. This detects the portion of exercising heart muscle that is receiving little or no blood through the narrowed coronary artery. The test is repeated at the end of the program, and if, at the same or a higher double product, the blood-starved area has shrunk, then the blood supply to the heart muscle must have increased, likely through the development of a collateral circulation.

A group of investigators from the Victoria Infirmary in Glasgow, Scotland, carried out just such a study on 40 men who suffered from angina. One year of exercise training, using the Royal Canadian Air Force 5BX plan, resulted in an average 34% reduction in the ischemic area. A report of a similar study from the University of Heidelberg in Germany, involving 18 patients who completed 12 months of vigorous exercise training and a low-fat diet, quoted a 54% reduction in exercise-induced ischemia.

Regression
Regression, or reversal of coronary atherosclerosis by shrinking the atheromatous deposit, was first demonstrated in rabbit studies in which atheromas induced by a high-fat diet gradually went away when a normal diet was reintroduced. The proof that regression could occur in human coronaries had to wait until the 1980s, when refinements in the technique of measuring the size of a deposit by coronary angiography were introduced. In 1987 Dr. David Blankenhorn and his colleagues from the University of Southern California demonstrated regression of coronary atherosclerosis in a small group of patients who were following a low-fat diet and taking a combination of the bile resin, colestipol, and niacin. Three years later Dr. Greg Brown and co-workers from the University of Washington reported similar results, the medication on this occasion being lovastatin (Mevacor). Both these reports spurred other investigators into action

to see if they could duplicate these findings. By and large, this proved to be the case. Mind you, while more patients in the treated groups were found to have regression than in the "usual care" control groups, not all those treated obtained such a favorable result.

You must realize that, over time, atherosclerosis can only do one of three things. It can get worse (and surely will if the risk factors that brought it about are not eliminated), it can stabilize, or it can regress. If we analyze the regression trials, we see that while some of the treated patients did indeed get worse, the majority either stabilized or showed some regression. Conversely, a significant number of the controls deteriorated, with only a small number stabilizing and even less regressing. Of course, it would be nice to know precisely why some of the treated got worse, but I'm afraid our present level of knowledge doesn't allow us to do that. However, the trials all show that the ability of the treatment to produce stability/regression depends on its capacity to reduce LDL-cholesterol and/or increase HDL-cholesterol.

The majority of the so-called regression trials to date have been drug trials, the commonest agent being one of the statins. However, Dr. Dean Ornish and his group from the University of California have described regression in a group of patients who followed his rehabilitation-type program that included a vegetarian diet, daily exercise, and stress-reduction techniques. The patients who adhered the most to his regimen obtained the greatest benefit, whereas those who complied the least did relatively poorly. Dr. Ornish did not attempt to identify which of the three strategies, the diet, the exercise, or the stress reduction therapy, was the most effective, and indeed all probably worked in concert. However, looking at the emphasis he places on each, it would be my judgment that the low-fat vegetarian diet plays the major role.

Dr. Gerhard Schuler and his colleagues from the

University Hospital in Heidelberg, Germany, also reported on a rehabilitation-type regression trial. His approach, however, was slightly different from that of Dr. Ornish. His patients followed the Step II American Heart Association low-fat diet (a daily allowance of 7% saturated fat from total calories and less than 200 mg of cholesterol) and an exercise program that consisted of 30 minutes of stationary cycling at home every day, as well as attendance at least twice a week at a 60-minute group workout in the gymnasium. At the end of a year, a high proportion of the treated patients showed stabilization and/or regression, in contrast to the controls, a higher percentage of whom got worse. One of Dr. Schuler's colleagues, Dr. Rainer Hambrecht, analyzed the data and found that exercise was the more effective of the two strategies in obtaining improvement. In fact, he was able to show that the patients who expended 2,000 or more kilocalories of energy a week (approximately five to six hours of exercise), obtained the most regression, those who expended about 1,500 kilocalories (three to four hours per week) the next, and those who expended around 1,000 kilocalories (less than three hours per week) the least. Just remember, however, that research must be applied to real life. Pragmatist that I am, I would advise both a low-fat diet and exercise training for the best results.

The possibility that the progression of atherosclerosis can be slowed or, in some cases even reversed, has given us more clues as to the nature of the disease. We now realize that reducing the high blood levels of cholesterol so often found in coronary heart disease stops the passage of cholesterol-laden scavenger cells into the plaque. This allows time for the cholesterol that has already penetrated the vessel wall to solidify and become more compact, and the fibrous cap that walls it off from the lumen to become thicker. The net result is a slightly smaller but eminently stable and less dangerous lesion.

But that is not all. One of the puzzles presented by the regression trials was the fact that patients suffering from angina obtained relief of their symptom quite early on in the trial, within a few weeks, and certainly before there was time for the changes I have just described to occur. How could this be? It seems the answer is to be found in the endothelium. Regression trials, whether they utilize a rigid low-fat diet, statin drugs, or exercise to improve the cholesterol profile, restore the ability of the endothelium to produce and secrete nitric oxide, and thus dilate the coronary arteries so as to allow a greater flow of blood to the heart muscle.

SECONDARY PREVENTION

So far we have seen that a rehabilitation program can greatly enhance the heart attack survivor's quality of life, improve functional capacity, counteract the risk factors for coronary heart disease, improve symptoms, and permit early return to work. For these reasons alone, in 1981 the Council on Scientific Affairs of the American Heart Association recommended that "cardiac rehabilitation should be considered as one of the treatments for coronary heart disease complementary to drug therapy or surgery". The following year the World Health Organization concurred, recommending "regular dynamic exercise as a rehabilitative measure in view of its effects on symptoms and work capacity, and risk factors."

In the final analysis, however, can we say that cardiac rehabilitation prevents a recurrent heart attack? From the outset, it has been the experience of all programs that recurrence rates are reduced. In a group of 2,500 post-coronary patients who had attended the Toronto program, a 10-year follow-up revealed an annual fatal recurrence rate of 1.9%. This compared very favorably with the annual rate of 3% to 4% reported for sedentary patients who had not been referred for exercise rehabilitation. However, we wanted to investigate the possibility that our results might have been biased by the fact that the physicians had chosen to refer to the program only those patients most likely to benefit and had excluded those who were the most ill. In order to do this, we matched patients according to their smoking habits, blood cholesterol levels, and presence or absence of angina, hypertension, and diabetes. We then compared those who continued to exercise regularly with those who stopped exercising for non-medical reasons such as boredom, being too busy, and general lack of motivation. Analysis of the data revealed that the death rate from recurrent heart attack was 60% lower in the exercisers over the ten-year period.

A number of prospective randomized exercise trials have been carried out during the 1970s and the 1980s in order to address the question of secondary prevention. All have shown a reduction in the incidence of recurrent fatal heart attack in the exercisers, but the results have not always reached statistically significant levels. The reason for this has been the inadequate number of subjects and the short period of follow-up, both the results of inadequate funding.

Given the problems of inadequate numbers and short follow-up that have typified the randomized exercise trials, the most reasonable approach has been to use meta-analysis. This was first carried out by Dr. Graham May and his colleagues, who pooled the data from a number of randomized trials and found a statistically significant 19% reduction in total mortality as a result of exercise training. Dr. Neil Oldridge and his co-workers from Ontario combined the results of ten randomized clinical trials and found a 25% reduction in recurrent fatal heart attacks in the exercising group.

In 1989 Dr. Gerald O'Connor and his colleagues published an analysis of 22 randomized trials, and found that exercise programs reduced the risk of fatal recurrence by 20% and the risk of sudden death by as much as 37%.

I think it is fair to say that we now have conclusive evidence that a carefully prescribed and supervised post-coronary exercise rehabilitation training program which includes behavior modification strategies to reduce cholesterol levels and eliminate smoking, as well as counteract obesity, diabetes, and hypertension, can play an important role in reducing fatal recurrence rates and sudden cardiac death.

11. Your Exercise Prescription

As a result of 30 years' experience training some 20,000 coronary heart disease patients at the Toronto Centre, we have developed a plan that, followed carefully and sensibly, will provide a safe and effective method of developing endurance fitness. However, let me start with a word of warning. Circumstances and individuals vary. Mindless adherence to this or any other training system could have unpleasant consequences, especially for those with coronary heart disease. While training usually leads to improved health and heart function, coronary disease can occasionally become unstable. The warning signs and symptoms of such deterioration are described on pages 264–265. If they become apparent, the exercise prescription should be reduced immediately. Similarly, if you have difficulty completing the prescribed workout, you should modify the requirements to suit your own tolerance. If in doubt, talk to your physician. *Prudence takes precedence over enthusiasm when you are training a damaged heart!* Accurate pacing is essential. Thus, you will need to use a stopwatch since you are timing to the nearest half-minute and, unless you are walking on a track, to measure the course in a car.

With these precautions in mind, let's take a closer look at the training tables reproduced in the appendices. They consist of three phases.

Phase Ia

The point at which you start your training depends on your fitness level, as determined by your maximum oxygen intake and your age. If your initial maximal oxygen intake (VO_2max) is less than 16 mL/kg per minute (and we will see later how to measure this yourself), you should carry out a preliminary phase that lasts for eight weeks. In addition, those who are overweight, have been sedentary for many years, or suffer from musculoskeletal problems such as low back pain or mild osteoarthritis in their knees or hips should also adhere to the eight-week breaking-in period—even though their initial fitness may be higher than the specified level. This phase progresses you from one to two miles over an eight-week period, the pace increasing from 30 minutes per mile to 23 minutes per mile.

Phase Ib

If your VO_2max is higher than 16 mL, your initial goal should be a 3-mile (5-kilometer) walk. The speed of the walk will be determined by your level of fitness. The 3 miles (5 kilometers) should be approached in stages: for two weeks, walk 1 mile (1.6 kilometers); for the next two weeks, walk 2 miles (3 kilometers); and finally, walk the 3 miles (5 kilometers), all at the prescribed speed. After that, you will progress to the next level by walking the 3-mile (5-kilometer) distance at a quicker pace.

Try to walk five times a week, with two days' rest. It's immaterial whether these rest days are taken together, or split. The choice is a matter of personal convenience.

If you are 60 or older, I would suggest that you make three miles in 45 minutes your goal. There is no need to progress beyond this level unless, of course, you have been a lifelong exerciser.

I should point out that the maximal oxygen intake levels used in Phase Ia were derived from exercise tests carried out at the Centre on patients suffering from coronary artery disease.

Phase II

In this phase, the intensity of the workout is slowly increased to a desired pace. If you are under the age of 45 and free from coronary heart disease or any of its manifestations, that pace is 10 minutes per mile (6 minutes per kilometer); if over 45 and under 60, or suffering from coronary heart disease or any of its manifestations, then that pace is 12 minutes per mile (7.5 minutes per kilometer). When you achieve your desired pace, the distance is lengthened to 4 miles (6.5 kilometers), at the same speed. This phase is crucial and may take many months to complete; if you suffer from coronary heart disease, you should be particularly alert for such adverse symptoms as chest pain, extreme breathlessness, irregular heart action, or light-headedness during the workout. If the condition of your heart is unstable, the instability is more likely to reveal itself at the quicker pace.

For most of us, walking at a pace quicker than 15 minutes per mile (9.5 minutes per kilometer) or 4 miles (6.5 kilometers) per hour is less economical and therefore more strenuous than jogging. To avoid this strain, short jogging segments are added to the training when the prescription calls for a 14.5 minutes-per-mile (9-minutes-per-kilometer) pace. This is done gradually through each of five stages until one attains a 12 minutes-per-mile (7.5-minutes-per kilometer) pace, at which time the entire distance of 3 miles (5 kilometers) is jogged (see Appendix B).

The jogging technique is described in detail later. At this stage it is sufficient to say that it should be relaxed, flat-footed and with short strides; the speed should be little above that of a walk. Actually, I think the term "plodding" is more descriptive than jogging.

Phase III
In Phase III, you progress to jogging 5 miles (8 kilometers) in 50 or 60 minutes, depending on your age and whether you are suffering from coronary heart disease. It takes about 12 months or more to reach this goal. Anyone who has managed to progress through the first two phases and is free from symptoms and signs should be able to finish Phase 3, but it should be undertaken only by those who really enjoy jogging. Jogging for an hour a day, five times a week is time-consuming and is not for everyone, but it pays off in a higher level of cardiorespiratory fitness. From the ranks of the "one-hour joggers" have come many postcoronary marathoners. Nonetheless, this phase is strictly optional.

HOW TO USE THE TABLES

Determining Your Starting Level
How fit are you? The only way to answer this accurately is to take a formal exercise test, which will measure your aerobic power, or maximal oxygen intake. The test will also indicate any electrocardiographic abnormalities that develop during training sessions. Such a test is mandatory for all patients entering my exercise rehabilitation program. If you are a would-be exerciser and have a heart problem, ask your physician to arrange an exercise test. If he or she doesn't do this procedure, ask to be referred to a physician who does.

If you have had a heart attack, or suffer from angina pectoris or palpitations and there are no facilities for exercise testing in your area, then to ensure your safety, start at the very beginning of the training tables, that is, at Level 1 of Phase Ia. Again, you should pursue this course *only if you have had prior clearance from your physician.*

If you are healthy and would like to determine your aerobic fitness level, your first step should be to complete the Physical Activity Readiness Questionnaire (see Appendix F). This was designed for use before taking the Canadian Standardized Test of Fitness, a similar submaximal bench test to the one about to be described. If you pass this questionnaire—that is, if you answer no to all the questions—then proceed as follows.

Submaximal Step Test
The following submaximal step test is one devised by Professor Roy Shephard, and I am indebted to him for its use here. The procedure requires you to step up and down two steps of 9 inches (23 centimeters) each, to a count of six. Keep your feet flat and stand up straight. Start with the feet together on the ground, then left foot on the first step—count one; right foot on the second step—count two; left foot joins right foot—count three; right foot on the first step—count four; left foot on the ground—count five; right foot joins left foot—count six. The lead leg can be alternated every other minute to reduce fatigue.

The rate of stepping is important since it affects the energy cost of the test. Our aim is an effort intensity about 75% of maximum. This will, of course, vary with age and body weight, and therefore Appendix G gives the appropriate tempo in terms of steps per minute, as well as the energy cost of this effort in milliliters of oxygen per kilogram per minute. The accompanying table also shows the 75% age-related anticipated heart rate after three minutes of stepping; this rate is based on the normal sedentary population and is accurate to within plus or minus ten beats per minute.

Once you have worked out the correct stepping rate

for your age and weight, practice with a stopwatch until you get the tempo, then step up and down for three minutes. Your aim is to attain your approximate target heart rate within that time. Immediately on stopping, take a ten-second pulse count (see pages 265–266 for instructions). With this figure, using the appropriate age-related nomogram (Appendix A), you can calculate your maximal oxygen intake.

A line joining your energy cost of stepping and your exercise heart rate will intersect the center line at your estimated maximal oxygen intake, expressed in milliliters of oxygen. Dividing this by your weight in kilograms (1 kilogram = 2.2 pounds) will give you your maximal oxygen intake expressed in milliliters of oxygen per kilogram per minute. Apply this figure to Phase Ib of the training tables, and you have your starting level of training.

Let us say you are a 50-year-old male who weighs 160 pounds (72 kilograms). Appendix G tells you to carry out the step test at the rate of 102 steps per minute to utilize 1,885 milliliters of oxygen per minute, which, for the average sedentary individual of that age and weight, would be equivalent to three-quarters of all-out effort. As a further check, the resultant pulse rate for that degree of effort (75% of maximum) is obtained from the accompanying table, i.e., 140 beats per minute.

You now carry out the test at the required rate of stepping for three minutes. At the end of this time you take your ten-second pulse count. Let us say it comes to 25 beats in 10 seconds, or 150 beats per minute. Then, from nomogram E you read off a predicted maximal oxygen intake of 2,200 milliliters per minute (a line joining 1,885 on the right column and 150 on the left column intersects the center sloping line at 2,200). You divide your predicted maximal oxygen intake of 2,200 by your weight in kilograms (72) and you obtain a $\dot{V}O_2$max corrected for weight of 30.3 mL/kg per minute. Applying this to the training tables would mean that you start at Level 7 of Phase Ib, or 3 miles (5 kilometers) in 45 minutes.

This might sound complicated but it is easier to do than to describe. However, if you find it a chore even to contemplate, then skip it and start at Phase Ia, Level 1.

Some Warnings
If you develop chest pain or discomfort, extreme breathlessness, light-headedness, or other adverse symptoms before the three minutes are up, stop immediately and note your pulse rate. It will represent your maximal heart rate for training purposes. For safety's sake, obtain your doctor's permission before you start the exercise program. If he or she agrees that exercise can help you, then start at the preliminary conditioning stage of the tables, and be sure that your pulse rate during the workout remains at least ten beats per minute below the symptom-producing level.

If after two minutes or so of stepping you feel that you cannot continue because your legs are too tired, stop. You are even less fit than the average sedentary person of your age and weight. If you take your pulse rate at the time that you have to stop, you will find that it is already well above the target rate. Don't despair, try again the following day, but this time choose the next lowest tempo listed in the table, e.g., 96 instead of 102 steps per minute.

Two very important points! Your stepping rate must be as accurately timed as possible. The best way to do this is to use a simple metronome, the sort that piano teachers use. Secondly, pulse rate should be obtained immediately on stopping. Ideally it should be taken during the last minute of the test, but this is very difficult to do. Instead, as you stop, take a ten-second pulse count, and then multiply the result by six to give a full minute's count. Remember, heart rate begins to drop rapidly with the cessation of exercise, and if you delay as little as even 30 seconds in finding and counting your pulse, the result will not truly represent your heart rate in the final minutes of the test.

Finally, at the risk of being unduly repetitive, let me once again warn you against attempting this or any other self-administered test without the permission of your physician—especially if you have any symptoms of coronary artery disease. Paradoxically, those most curious to know their fitness level are the overweight, sedentary, obviously unfit members of the population—precisely those in whom atherosclerosis is likely to be present. Beware that curiosity doesn't kill the fat cat.

Taking Your Pulse Count
It is essential that you take your pulse accurately. As the beating heart ejects its blood into the aorta, the impulse is transmitted down the aorta's walls to all of its branches, where it is felt as a pulse. Thus, the pulse rate coincides with the heart rate. Physicians traditionally measure heart rate by timing the pulse of the radial artery, which is felt in the front of the wrist just below the base of the thumb. At this point the radial artery lies just beneath the skin and is easily felt because it can be steadied against the underlying wrist bones. Exercise physiologists tend to use the carotid pulse, the large artery in the front of the neck, which can be felt on either side of the Adam's apple; this vessel pumps very vigorously during exercise, and for that reason is easier to obtain.

Use whichever you find the easiest. If you use the carotid, however, be careful not to press too hard, otherwise you will press on a structure known as the carotid sinus, which will slow the heart rate momentarily. The advantage of taking the carotid pulse is that it allows you to operate a stopwatch in the other hand and so get an accurate count. If you are having difficulty in feeling the carotid pulse, you may be throwing your head back, a movement that causes the carotid arteries to move away from the front of the neck. If you want to feel the carotid pulse easily, then hold your head in the normal position, or even tilt it slightly forward.

Since you are counting for only ten seconds and multiplying by six, accuracy is essential. For uniformity's sake, we tell our patients to start counting "zero, one, two, three," etc., the zero marking the commencement of the ten-second count.

Why count for only ten seconds? Ideally, we want to know what the heart rate is *during* the exercise session. As soon as you start to work out, your resting heart rate climbs, and within two or three minutes reaches a plateau that remains steady for as long as you exercise—provided, of course, that you maintain the same pace. It is impractical to take the pulse rate while jogging, or even walking, but for 10 or 15 seconds after you stop your heart rate will remain at the plateau. Pulse rates, then, taken within ten seconds of stopping jogging or brisk walking, are a fairly accurate measure of the heart rate during the workout. Thereafter, the rate drops off rapidly. If you wait for even as short a time as 20 seconds to take your count, it will no longer be representative of the rate during exercise.

When to Move from One Phase to the Next

The tables are designed to train you at an intensity of approximately 50% to 70% of your maximal oxygen intake or, expressed another way, 60% to 80% of your maximal heart rate. As you become fitter, however, both your resting and your exercising pulse rates will become slower. Eventually, the intensity and duration of the prescribed workout will no longer obtain the required training pulse rate. When this stage is reached, progression to a higher level is indicated. Use nomogram A to determine this point. To use this nomogram, you need to know your resting and exercise pulse rates. Your maximal heart rate has already been estimated from age-related tables. Your resting pulse rate is taken immediately on awakening in the morning and before you get out of bed or after sitting relaxed in an armchair for five minutes or so.

When the prescribed walk/jog consistently fails to achieve the progressing pulse rate for a period of two weeks, then the time has come to move up to the next level of the table. Say, for instance, that a 40-year-old woman who started at Level 5, Phase Ib (3 miles or 4.8 kilometers in 48 minutes) had a resting pulse rate of 72 beats per minute. To use nomogram A, she would take a piece of dark thread and place one end at 72 on the resting heart rate column (values less than 72 can, for the purposes of prediction, be ignored). She would then stretch the thread to the 40 on the age column. The point where the thread crosses the center line is her progressing heart rate: 130 beats per minute. Thus, when her pulse count in the ten seconds following her 3-mile (4.8-kilometer) walk is at or below this level of 130 consistently for a period of two weeks (an average of ten successive workouts), she would be ready to progress to Level 6 (3 miles or 4.8 kilometers in 45 minutes). The use of the nomogram, therefore, enables safe and effective progression without constant retesting. It gives an element of objectivity to the training regime; instead of stepping up your program because you feel fit and well, you can apply a physiological measure to validate your enthusiasm.

To get maximal value from the nomogram, you must use it correctly. Not only must the exercise pulse rate be at or below the progressing heart rate *consistently* for ten or more exercise sessions, but progression to a higher level of effort should not be attempted if you are experiencing any of the signs of overtraining such as excessive tiredness, palpitations (premature ventricular beats), or muscle aches and pains. Your pulse rate must be charted at the end of each exercise session in order to keep an accurate record.

Of course, the nomogram contains two other variables, age and resting pulse rate. The majority of people reach the end of Phase II within a one- to two-year period; therefore, once you have started on the program, it should not be necessary to change your age level on the left-hand column. As for resting pulse rate, this also drops with training, but the change is more variable than with exercise pulse rate. For patients on a supervised program, a new resting pulse rate can be established at the time of each laboratory exercise test; failing this, it is a good idea to check your resting pulse rate every three to six months and adjust the right-hand column accordingly.

If You Suffer from Angina
So far, we have been discussing the use of the nomogram to check the progress of the individual who does not suffer from symptoms such as angina pectoris. What of the patient who suffers from symptoms, especially when exercising? For this individual, there is a special nomogram. Into this category also fall those patients whose formal exercise test revealed the presence of such ECG abnormalities as ST segment depression, exercise-induced frequent extrasystoles (see page 272), or some other complication (see Appendix A).

A hospital-type program with regular exercise testing can determine the exact level of exertion at which cardiac problems develop. Such repeated testing may be impractical, however, in a home program. A more individualized approach has therefore been developed that takes into account the pulse rate at which untoward symptoms or signs develop. Nomogram B permits the choice of a suitable starting level of exercise for the patient with symptoms and assures his or her subsequent safe progress through the various stages of the tables.

To use this nomogram, note must be made of the pulse rate at which the symptoms developed during an exercise test, either carried out in the doctor's office or at home. This is the maximum heart rate, symptom limited, or maxHR$_{SL}$. Using this figure, together with the resting pulse rate (obtained as previously), the training pulse rate can be read from nomogram B.

A word of warning: If the difference between your resting pulse rate and your maxHR$_{SL}$ is 40 beats per minute or less, you should exercise only under the strict supervision of a physician. As you can see from the nomogram, the spread between training and progressing heart rates would be small in your case, requiring careful, accurate professional monitoring.

If this proviso does not apply to you, a trial 1-mile (1.6-kilometer) walk is then taken, at a pace that is considered brisk, but not so fast as to bring on chest pain, skipped beats, or undue breathlessness. The pulse rate is taken in the ten seconds immediately following the walk and is compared with the desired training pulse rate. Depending on the result, the pace is adjusted to the nearest appropriate level in Phase Ib. Always err on the side of safety: keep the intensity of exercise below the level at which symptoms develop. It may take one or two sessions to select the desired pace, but with patience and care, it is surprising how accurate one can be.

The following example will illustrate the method. Assume you have a resting heart rate of 72 beats per minute. While being tested, you develop evidence of myocardial ischemia, say chest pain, at a heart rate of 124 beats per minute. This means you have a maxHR$_{SL}$ of 124. From the nomogram, you determine that your training heart rate$_{SL}$ is 110 beats per minute. You now go for a trial 1-mile (1.6-kilometer) walk, choosing a level course, and keeping the pace slow enough to avoid chest pain or undue breathlessness. At the end of the measured mile (1.6 kilometers), which took you 20 minutes to cover, your immediate postexercise pulse rate is 108 beats per minute. This, then, is your starting level (Level 1, Phase Ib for the under-45-year-old). Over the next six weeks, you will progress to 2 miles (3.2 kilometers) and then to 3 miles (4.8 kilometers), keeping the same pace of 20 minutes per mile (12.5 minutes per kilometer). Using the same nomogram, you can also tell what your progressing pulse rate should be (in this example, 100 beats per minute). After each workout, you chart your pulse rate, and when this consistently fails to achieve 100 beats per minute for ten consecutive sessions, and provided you have none of the adverse symptoms mentioned above, then you progress to Level 2, Phase Ib.

I feel that complicated cases should be exercise-tested every three months or so in order to have an objective measurement of improvement. When they can complete a test without adverse signs or symptoms, they can proceed in accordance with nomogram A. Complicated cases require much closer physician supervision than uncomplicated ones, and the individuals ideally should be enrolled in a formal postcoronary exercise rehabilitation class where they can be watched during supervised exercise sessions and monitored frequently during the workouts.

In the early stages, the individual with symptoms during exercise will progress at a slower rate than his or her symptomless colleagues. This is to be expected and should not be allowed to cause discouragement or depression. Above all, any temptation to progress faster than the tables indicate should be vigorously resisted. You cannot bully a damaged heart. This is one game where breaking the rules may mean more than the loss of a few yards or a few points; it may mean "game over" for the only player involved—yourself! So, have patience, and remember that if it took 20 years to get out of shape, you can't really expect to regain your fitness in a few months.

If You Are Taking Medication
Individuals who are taking a beta-blocker may have resting heart rates in the low fifties, with an accompanying reduction in heart rate at all levels of exertion, up to and

including maximum. Therefore, attempts to achieve heart rates, either during exercise testing or workouts, based on age-related tables may be disastrous. For this reason, I place all patients taking a beta-blocker in the complicated category and use nomogram B for establishing both training heart rate and progressing heart rate. We have found this procedure to work well and have demonstrated repeatedly that patients who are taking beta-blockers can obtain a significant training effect. Of course, as they develop a training bradycardia (slow heart rate), their resting and working heart rates drop, and this reduction may be increased by the effect of the medication. Rather than having the resting heart rate become too slow, we customarily wait until it reaches the forties and then request the patient's cardiologist to consider reducing the beta-blocker dosage. This usually results in a return of the resting rate to the mid or high fifties. As training continues, the rate eventually returns to the forties again, and once more the dosage may be reduced. Eventually the medication may be stopped altogether or may be continued in small doses for its secondary preventive effect.

Ideally, patients on a beta-blocker should try to exercise at approximately the same time each day. This will ensure that the blood levels of the medication are approximately the same during each workout, and therefore pulse rates will be stable.

Since beta-blockers relieve angina by reducing the Rate Pressure Product for a given level of effort, and since exercise training seems to produce the same result by way of the same mechanism, I am sometimes asked, "Why exercise? Why not just use the drug to get fit?" Apart from the fact that exercise training has fewer contraindications and side effects, the beta-blocker lowers *maximal* heart rate and blood pressure and so, unlike exercise training, may limit physical performance. Of course, where angina is preventing everyday submaximal levels of activity, relief by a beta-blocker can for all practical purposes enhance physical capacity.

Calcium channel blockers do not interfere with the training effect, and they are mentioned here primarily because of their effect on pulse rate. Adalat and Cardene, the most commonly used for hypertension, will frequently increase pulse rate, and for this reason may often be given in conjunction with a beta-blocker. Cardizem slows pulse rate, although not as dramatically as the beta-blockers. Finally, Isoptin either has no effect or reduces pulse rate.

Digitalis is a drug that often reduces the resting pulse rate, but in the dosages usually given does not have much effect on the working or maximum pulse level. For this reason, it does not interfere with a training effect, although allowance must be made for the fact that it can produce a resting bradycardia, which should not be confused with the effects of training.

If You Are Suffering from Skipped Beats

When you take your pulse, you are counting your heart *rate*. At the same time, you are also noting the heart rhythm and how regular it is. The commonest form of irregularity is one in which there appears to be a missed or *skipped* beat. This can be alarming to the novice pulse taker, who may think that the heart has actually dropped a beat or, if the pause is sufficiently long, may imagine that the heart has actually stopped beating. If you know that one of the medical terms for a skipped beat is a *premature* beat (or extrasystole), you are more likely to be reassured.

Let us take a look at what happens during the cardiac cycle. During the period of systole, blood is ejected into the aorta by the powerful muscular left ventricle. This is felt throughout the arteries of the body as the pulse. During the period of diastole that follows, both right and left ventricles are relaxed, and blood flows back from the body and the lungs through the atria into the ventricles again. If a heartbeat occurs prematurely, the period of diastole is shortened, and therefore less blood enters the ventricles. This in turn means that the volume of blood ejected during the following period of systole is also reduced and may not even be sufficient to transmit a palpable impulse to the carotid or radial arteries: thus the "skipped" beat. Nevertheless, the fact that you cannot feel the pulse should not alarm you into thinking that the heart has failed to beat; in fact, the beat has occurred, but earlier than expected.

Why do skipped, or premature, beats occur? A clue to the answer lies in the other medical term for skipped beats. They are also known as *ectopic* beats. Ectopic comes from the Greek meaning "away from the place." The normal signal for a heartbeat originates in a button of specialized tissue (the sinoatrial node) located in the upper corner of the right atrium (Figure 36). From there, 72 times every minute, the signal spreads through the walls of the top of the heart to reach a receiver, another collection of specialized cells, situated between the atria and the ventricles at the top of the intraventricular septum (the atrioventricular [AV] node). From the AV node, the signal then proceeds down the intraventricular septum by way of two tracks known as the right and left bundles, and finally ascends the walls of both ventricles. Once its journey is complete, the ventricles contract and the heartbeat occurs. You will remember that the passage of this signal is charted electrically on the electrocardiogram; the P wave represents the start of the message from the SA node (or, if you wish to think of it in football terms, the quarterback) through the atria to the AV node (or receiver) and the QRS deflection marks the completion of the signal (or play) through the bundles (or lines).

Because the heart is such a vital organ, it has a number of built-in safeguards to ensure that it continues to work in spite of any number of malfunctions. If, for instance, our

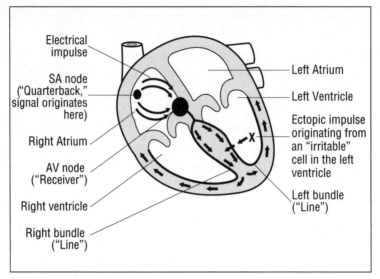

Figure 36: How the Heart Beats
The electrical signal starts in the SA node, passes to the AV node, and then travels along both right and left bundles. An ectopic impulse, causing a premature beat, is also shown.

quarterback, the SA node, who is programmed to fire a pass 72 times a minute, is injured, that does not mean that play cannot commence. The AV node, or receiver, is programmed to fire at the rate of 64 times per minute. If, after waiting a suitable period of time, it fails to receive a signal from the SA node, it initiates its own, sending it down both lines to complete the journey as usual and trigger the next heartbeat. But what if our receiver, the AV node, is injured? Is it game over? Not on your life (no pun intended). Heart muscle cells are unique. They are all endowed with the property we refer to as automaticity. It means that, when the need arises, they can automatically take the place of the SA node; that is, they are all potential quarterbacks. The cells in the ventricles are programmed to fire at the rate of 32 beats per minute. If signals are not received from the SA node or the AV node, then, again after waiting an appropriate period of time, they can fire a signal to any part of the right or left bundle below the AV node, set the line in action, and make sure that the ventricles contract. A signal coming from one of these cells originates in an area away from its rightful place, the SA node, and is therefore referred to as being ectopic in origin.

Why do ectopic or premature ventricular beats occur? Some individuals have ventricular muscle heart cells that are overly ambitious to become quarterbacks. These are the "race horse" types. When their adrenaline is flowing, their heart cells are all "fired up," too impatient to await the orderly sequence of play, and so one of them fires off a signal prematurely. Since they are located closer to the conducting bundles than the SA node, their signal arrives first and is often well on its way even before the AV node is activated. Thus, the premature beat occurs very shortly after the prior normal beat. At the same time, both SA and AV nodes, recognizing that they have been forestalled, abort their own signals and wait for the next cardiac cycle to start. Because the ectopic beat is premature, there appears to be a longer pause, or skip, occurring before the next normal beat. In fact, the time interval between the normal beat, the premature beat, and the next normal beat is the same as that which would occur between three normal beats. However, because the premature beat is not felt at the pulse, it seems that a very lengthy pause has occurred.

Some individuals' heart cells are susceptible to stimulants such as caffeine (tea, coffee, cola drinks, chocolate), cigarette smoke, excessive alcohol (usually spirits), stressful circumstances that lead to the release of adrenaline and noradrenaline, fatigue, or, in the case of coronary artery disease, shortage of blood supply to the heart muscle. Most people experience isolated skipped beats from time to time, but when they become frequent (every second, third, or fourth beat), are aggravated by physical exertion, and are found in the presence of known coronary artery disease, then they should be reported to the physician before regular exercise training is undertaken. Various techniques for obtaining ambulatory electrocardiogram tracings are now available, and these can often pinpoint the precise source of the ectopic cell. The decision can then be taken as to whether they need to be suppressed by medication or surgery.

The medical profession has gone through a series of changes of thinking with regard to the treatment of skipped beats. In the First World War, an irregular heartbeat was considered to be a sign of cardiac disease, and if it was detected in the young conscript or draftee, he was labelled with the rather vague diagnosis of D.A.H. (disordered action of the heart) and rejected for service. However, by the Second World War it was recognized that, in the absence of proven heart disease, episodes of irregular heart action were quite common in young men of draft age. Indeed, many of these individuals flew bombers and fighter planes in the Royal Canadian Air Force throughout the war, and a follow-up into their sixties and seventies showed that their subsequent incidence of heart disease was no different from individuals who were free from skipped beats. As the epidemic of coronary disease spread in the postwar period, and with the development of sophisticated electrocardiogram monitoring techniques, once again cardiac irregularities began to be seen in the coronary care units in association with heart attacks. At the same time, new drugs appeared on the scene that were capable of suppressing these extra beats. However, it should be pointed out that these drugs have side effects, and considerable judgment and skill must be exercised by the physician who prescribes them.

In very recent years there has been a tendency to use less drug medication, based on the realization that many types of skipped beats, or arrhythmias as they are known, are not life-threatening. In general, they have to be quite frequent and accompanied by symptoms such as blackouts or fainting before being considered for treatment by antiarrhythmic drugs.

12. Exercise Do's and Don'ts

Don't Expect Miracles

A few basic facts about physical fitness should be borne in mind. First, each of us has an optimal level of endurance fitness appropriate for our age and genetic background. Once we reach that level, more intensive training will result in only marginal gains. Unfortunately, few if any of us even come close to our optimal level. The training tables in Appendix B have been devised to help you achieve a level of fitness that is suitable for your age and general tolerance. They are based on maximum oxygen intake levels attained by patients on our postcoronary exercise program and should, therefore, be well within the capabilities of the vast majority of readers. Of course, there are always exceptions to the rule. For example, some people will be unable to progress to the end of Phase II. They may stick at an earlier level because of adverse symptoms, failure to achieve the progressing heart rate, or excessive fatigue after the workout. Does this mean that they are wasting their time training? Certainly not. It simply means that they have attained their appropriate duration and intensity of workout, and if they continue to train at this level, they will maintain their optimal fitness.

There is a misapprehension about the development of fitness that is important to dispel. Most people believe that a training program, carried out regularly, results in a gradual day-by-day improvement in their physical state. If you are expecting to progress in this manner, you will be disappointed. What usually happens is that you work away for weeks, or even months, without any apparent change, and then suddenly one day, you find the pre-scribed training session quite easy. At the same time, you notice that your postworkout pulse rate has dropped a few beats or more. When the same thing happens on the next workout, you will realize that you have suddenly and almost miraculously attained a new level of fitness.

What is the explanation? One of the major effects of training is to open up new blood capillaries in the skele-tal muscle tissue so as to transport more oxygen to the working cells. These new capillaries, so small that they can be seen only under a microscope, do not form gradually. They "open up," almost like a budding flower seen under time-lapse photography, in response to the stimulus of repeated and prolonged training sessions. The duration of their formative period varies from individual to individ-ual, but the "plateau" between periods of increased cap-illarization is an essential part of the process. Don't become discouraged because your condition appears to be stationary. In fact, the preliminary work of capillarization is continuing; the next day or week may see the great leap forward.

Do Jog in the Correct Manner
Recreational jogging for fun and fitness is reputed to have started in New Zealand in the 1960s. It was introduced by the world-famous track coach Arthur Lydiard, who believed in long, slow, distance training for his competi-tive runners, even his half-milers and milers.

Despite its long history, the technique of jogging is

still a mystery to some. It differs from running only in its speed of progression. In our context, jogging means running at a pace no quicker than 10 minutes per mile (6 minutes per kilometer) or for our coronary patients, 12 minutes per mile (7.5 minutes per kilometer). The action is simple; take short steps, and land flat-footed. The body should be erect, the shoulders and neck relaxed, and the head held naturally (if you fix your eyes on an imaginary spot about 30 yards (27 meters) ahead, this will give the correct head inclination). The elbows should be bent not quite to a right angle, so that the hands move backward and forward easily about the level of the hips; the more you bend your elbows, the shorter the lever made by the arms, and the faster they will swing back and forth. As any sprinter will tell you, pumping your arms vigorously will automatically increase leg speed; so use an easy relaxed arm motion. The short stride and the flat-foot landing will ensure that your center of gravity remains over the leading foot, thus preventing too much of a forward body lean, which is all very well for the competitive middle-distance runner, but plays no part in recreational jogging.

Do Buy the Right Equipment
You will need a stopwatch for counting your pulse and also timing your workout. Most models on the market today are relatively cheap and accurate. However, there is not much point in having an accurate stopwatch if you haven't carefully measured the distance you are walking or jogging. If you are working out on the road, you will get an accurate enough reading from a car odometer; I have rarely found these to be misleading—unless, of course, the hot rodder in the family has fitted your sedan with outsize tires!

Shoes are the most important piece of equipment, and you should not attempt to economize here. Just think of the number of times your feet will strike the ground when you are jogging five hours a week, week in, week out. Your feet need to be protected, and it is precisely for this reason that special shoes have been designed for the jogger. Although each manufacturer has individual variations, the following features tend to be common to all. They are quite light, a pair usually weighing less than 2 pounds (1 kilogram). The sole is flexible, but thick enough to absorb shock. It is laminated with cushioning layers of foam (or encapsulated air bags) for shock absorption, and high-duty carbon rubber for stability and durability. An arch support is built in, and the lining of the tongue specially padded to protect the instep from the pressure of the laces. The upper is made of nylon, and the portion around the heel (the counter) is reinforced so as to grip the heel firmly and prevent it from wobbling from side to side as you run. Since the heel takes most of our body weight when we run, a special rubber heel wedge is often a feature and, to protect the Achilles tendon, or heel cord, the back of the shoe is reinforced with padding that adds support and prevents chafing.

Needless to say, no one shoe is ideal. Find the particular brand of running shoe that suits you best. In recent years, an incredible number of excellent jogging shoes have appeared on the market, and most sports outfitters will carry an extensive supply. Many of the sales clerks are experts and can help you obtain the right fit and style for your body build and weight.

Do Wear Comfortable Clothes

A *sweat suit* is valuable, but not essential for walking or jogging. A pair of comfortable pants and a sweater will do just as well. Unless you live in Florida or Southern California, much of your training will be done in some form of garb that covers your legs and upper body. A commercial sweat suit is probably the most convenient. My personal prefer-ence is for one made from a mixture of nylon and cotton, since it absorbs the sweat much better than a pure nylon suit. Some synthetic materials, such as Gore-Tex, are particularly good at protecting you from the rain or wind. Running shorts and T-shirt complete the list, but neither represents much of a strain on the budget. While some joggers like to avoid socks, the majority prefer a light cotton pair in order to prevent blisters. Vigorously exercising women should consider a specially constructed sports bra.

Don't Overtrain
The art of scientific training is to apply just enough overload, or physical stress, to achieve the desired result while at the same time avoiding overstrain and breakdown. Although overtraining is more likely to occur in the competitive athlete than in the fun jogger, nevertheless the coronary-prone individual has a fine margin of error and should recognize the signs and symptoms of excess.

Be alert, therefore, for such signs as excessive muscle soreness, an increase in your resting pulse rate, or undue tiredness persisting to the next training session. Angina is a sympton, of course, but increased palpitations (skipped beats), marked breathlessness, or light-headedness during an exercise session can also be evidence of shortage of blood to the heart muscle, and their consistent presence during exercise suggests that the coronary blood flow is unable to keep pace with the other training responses. Do not proceed to the next training level if they are present. If they appear for the first time, or become more frequent in response to an exercise prescription, stop your training program and consult your physician.

However, before blaming the prescription entirely for increase in symptoms, consider whether you are under unusual stress at work or are working prolonged hours. Typically, postcoronary exercisers are enthusiastic and conscientious and often try to maintain the prescribed level of exercise even during busy spells at their job. The result is that when they are at work they worry that they won't have time to carry out their exercise prescription, while during their workout they worry that the time spent in training could have been spent at work. I have learned to beware of various occupations at certain times of the year: for instance, accountants at income tax time, and department store workers during the Christmas season. At these times of stress, the regular exercise prescription may give rise to angina, especially at the end of a long and worrisome day. The obvious solution is to cut back the exercise prescription until the work pattern returns to normal.

If the high stress on the job looks as if it is going to be permanent, you might reduce the level of training. But, in the long run, you would do better to take a serious look at the job itself and your attitude toward it. Are you giving more to your job than your employer expects? Are you trying to carry out a job for which you lack the necessary aptitude? An honest answer to these questions may be very revealing.

Perhaps you should also examine your sleep habits. Chronic lack of sleep seems to be a feature of modern urban living. The long journey home from the office to the suburbs usually means a late evening meal, often followed by watching television. The occasional late night is inevitable, but don't make a habit of it and expect to reap the benefits of training. And don't assume the running program is making you feel overly tired when you haven't bothered to adjust your sleep pattern so as to allow for the additional energy expenditure.

For those who are hooked on exercise, and are jogging 5 miles (8 kilometers) in an hour, the recognition of overtraining may be difficult. The explanation lies in Dr. Hans Selye's famous theory of stress. The application of mild and healthful stress changes the body's mechanism to make it more resistant to that particular form of stress, and it also produces a feeling of elation and euphoria, which may last for some hours after the stress has been applied. However, if the stress, or in our case, training stimulus, is continued to excessive levels, then specific resistance develops at the cost of generalized resistance. In other words, the highly trained runner becomes extremely resistant to the fatigue of running, but less and less resistant to concurrent infections or mental stress. This is probably the explanation for the high susceptibility of world-class athletes to food poisoning, dysentery, or the sort of flu-like viruses that often rampage through athletes' training camps. In any event, while the loss of generalized resistance may be obvious to a trained observer such as a sports medicine physician or coach, it is often hidden from the athlete by the short-lived sense of well-being that follows each training session. Thus, he or she may be losing weight, becoming more irritable, and developing many of the other symptoms described above; but each time he works out he feels great for two or three hours, and so falls into the trap of repeating the training sessions in the hope that his overall condition will improve. Again, this problem is less common in the fun jogger who is exercising for health, but may be applicable for those who get more seriously involved.

Do Pay Attention to Your Body's Response
In the initial stages of the exercise program, and particularly if you have been sedentary for years, it is inevitable that you will develop mild pain and discomfort in the legs, Achilles tendonitis or inflammation of your heel cord, sore feet, and other relatively minor muscle, tendon, and ligamentous injuries that follow a regimen of walking and jogging after years of inactivity. Although not serious, they are a nuisance and can have an adverse effect on your motivation. A careful warm-up, including stretching, can help, but once again if the problem persists throughout a

complete workout, or is felt between the workouts, then a complete rest is indicated. Usually a week is sufficient, but if the trouble recurs on returning to exercise at the end of that time, see your physician, who will probably prescribe a course of physiotherapy. Close adherence to the tables, as well as to the technique of jogging previously described, will reduce such injuries to a minimum. The Toronto Centre's incidence of injuries over the years has been negligible, despite the fact that we deal almost entirely with middle-aged sedentary individuals who haven't exercised for years.

A pleasant feeling of physical relaxation and tiredness should follow a suitable workout. In many cases, there is an immediate postexercise sense of exhilaration (for this reason, some people prefer to work out in the morning or early evening rather than just prior to going to bed). Excessive fatigue may be defined as tiredness that is still present after a good night's sleep. It generally responds to three or four days' rest from exercise.

Usually after a workout, the pulse returns to its resting level within two hours; this may take a little longer on a hot and humid day. However, a rapid heart rate (tachycardia) that persists for four hours or longer suggests that the workout has been too intense.

If you find that you are dreading your next workout, this is another sure sign of overtraining. A fit individual usually looks forward to the exercise session, either as a relief from workday tensions or out of sheer animal spirits. In the early stages of the program, you may not be quite this enthusiastic, but you shouldn't actively dislike the thought of training. If you do, then the exercise prescription is too ambitious and should be reduced.

Don't Continue to Exercise If You Suffer from Angina
If you suffer chest pain on exertion, then you should slow your pace until the pain goes away. If the pain does not

subside within 100 yards (91 meters) or so, then stop, and wait for it to disappear. As soon as this happens, start to walk again, but at a slower pace. Some individuals can "walk through" their angina, but I caution against this in the early stages of the program until you have become thoroughly familiar with your exercise response.

On occasions, your physician may advise you to take a tablet of nitroglycerine or some similar medication during the workout in order to relieve the angina. Alternatively, you may be asked to take the medication ten minutes or so before your training session in order to prevent the onset of angina. I am frequently asked if this use of nitroglycerine in some way reduces the effectiveness of the training. The answer is no. The fact that it enables you to complete your exercise session is, in itself, proof of its value. As you become more fit, you will find that the angina occurs less and less frequently, until eventually you are able to carry out a full workout without the necessity of medication.

If your angina is so severe that you cannot walk or jog continuously for the prescribed time, don't despair; you can use another training method I have found to be very effective. This is known as interval training; in its modified form, it consists of walking for 15 to 30 seconds at a pace just below that which brings on the chest discomfort. Stroll casually for a further minute, and then repeat the walk for another 15 to 30 seconds. In this way, cover a mile (1.6 kilometers), always staying below the level of effort that brings on the pain. You will eventually find that you can extend the distance to 2 or 3 miles (3 to 5 kilometers) in this way, with only infrequent episodes of discomfort.

Don't Exercise after Meals or on an Empty Stomach
Exercise should never be carried out within two hours of eating a heavy meal. This rule is particularly important for

angina sufferers, since the digestion of food requires an extra supply of blood to the intestines, thus depleting the coronary circulation. In a situation where the coronary arteries are already narrowed, the loss of even a small reservoir of blood in this area can give rise to myocardial ischemia.

If you are an early-morning jogger, remember that after eight or ten hours of sleep your blood sugar is very low, and you should not exercise on a completely empty stomach. Have a roll and a glass of orange juice before sallying forth.

Do Warm Up

Angina often occurs during the early part of the workout and can frequently be prevented by a warm-up. This means spending five to ten minutes doing simple calisthenics, or walking at a pace slower than the prescribed intensity, until your body breaks into a light sweat. As soon as the sweat appears, you are warmed up and may commence your prescription. This is very important for those who suffer from angina and frequently is as effective as taking a nitroglycerine tablet. If your prescription is still at a low level, then you can enhance your warm-up at even slower speeds by wearing a sweater under your track suit to accelerate the onset of the stage of perspiration.

Do Cool Down

Exercise deaths are rare, but when they do occur it is often at the termination of the exercise session, or even on the way to the locker room. Often a careful evaluation of the circumstances will reveal that the unfortunate victim suffered from previously unrecognized coronary disease, had stopped the workout suddenly, and failed to cool down. The suggested mechanism is as follows: Physical effort involves the delivery of a high volume of oxygenated blood to the working muscles and the equally fast return of the deoxygenated blood to the right side of the heart. This return is accelerated by the massaging action of the contracting muscles on their deep veins. If the exerciser stops suddenly, the heart continues to deliver the same volume of blood for the next few seconds, but the pumping action of the muscles ceases, blood pools in the limbs, and there is a sudden drop in the return flow. The result is an equally precipitous drop in the amount of blood ejected in the following heartbeats. Blood pressure falls and coronary blood flow is reduced. This situation in itself can compromise the circulation to the heart muscle.

However, there is further adverse mechanism at work involving changes in the "fight or flight" stress hormones, adrenaline and noradrenaline. Both of these substances, particularly the latter, circulate throughout the body in high concentrations during physical exercise, ensuring that blood pressure and heart rate keep pace with the demand of the working muscles for an enhanced blood supply. With sudden cessation of exercise and blood pooling, the consequent sharp drop in blood pressure is interpreted by the brain as a failure in the blood delivery system, with the result that there is an immediate release of even greater quantities of noradrenaline in order to correct the situation. From animal studies, we know that if we suddenly expose atherosclerotic hearts to abnormally high concentrations of noradrenaline, we can induce irregular beats, tachycardia, ventricular fibrillation, and cardiac arrest. The lesson, then, is obvious. Spend five or ten minutes winding down after your exercise session, moving around and gradually letting your body return to its resting level.

While on the topic, a caution should be sounded against having hot showers immediately after a workout. A significant proportion of blood flow has already been diverted to the muscles. A hot shower dilates the blood vessels of the skin, further reducing the flow through the coronary circulation. This situation, following an exercise session, may prove too much for the individual with coronary artery disease. So I advise all my patients to wait 10 or 15 minutes after exercising before taking a lukewarm shower.

Do Choose a Flat Course

Hill running may be great training for competitive athletes, but it should be avoided by middle-aged joggers. It will certainly aggravate a tendency to angina, since the energy expended in running up a slope can be considerable. All of the distances listed in the tables are assumed to be on a flat course. Ideally, therefore, all of your workouts should be on the flat. If hills are unavoidable, then reduce your speed accordingly so as to achieve the same heart rate and/or rating of perceived exertion on the Borg scale you associate with your usual course.

Do Beware Summer Heat

Your body temperature results from a combination of heat generated by your working muscles and internal organs and heat absorbed from the surrounding air. As you sit reading this book, presumably relaxed and calm, you are generating about 75 calories of heat every hour. If you were to put the book down (not yet, please), stand up and go for a 3-mile (5-kilometer) walk, you would generate about 300 calories an hour.

If the body had no means of dissipating its internal heat, your temperature would rise about 2°F (1°C) an hour, even under the resting conditions; under moderate working conditions, the rise would be in the order of 9°F (5°C) an hour. Like any other machine, the body has a temperature at which all the various parts function most efficiently, 98.6°F (37°C). If the temperature of the body climbs above 110°F (43°C) or falls below 84°F (29°C), essential organs such as the heart, kidneys, and liver cease to work, and death becomes imminent. But since, as we have seen, even staying alive generates enough heat to kill us in a matter of hours, we must have a very efficient mechanism for dissipating this excess heat and holding the body temperature consistently close to the 98.6°F (37°C) level. How does this system work?

Physical exercise results in the shunting of as much as a gallon (3.8 liters) of blood through the blood vessels of the muscles every minute. Since these muscles are working, their internal temperature is raised, and this heats the blood that passes through them. The heated blood then returns to the heart, where it is pumped around the body again. As it flows through the brain, it triggers off the Benzinger reflex, a mechanism by which the blood vessels to the skin are opened up and the sweat glands are stimulated to work overtime. Warm blood can now dissipate its heat into the surrounding *cooler* air by the processes of convection, conduction, and radiation. Notice I said *cooler* air—that is, an air temperature lower than the skin temperature of 92°F (33°C). What happens when the air temperature is high, approaching that of the skin? Under these circumstances, the body has to depend more and more on the evaporation of sweat to lower the body temperature. The mere act of sweating has no cooling effect per se; it is the vaporization, or evaporation of the sweat from the surface of the body that is all important.

There is a limit to the rate at which one can sweat. In the average unconditioned individual this amounts to about 1 quart (1 liter) per hour; in a trained, heat-acclimatized exerciser, this figure may be increased to as much as 1 gallon (3.8 liters) per hour. Evaporation of sweat can also be influenced by a number of physical conditions. If the air is humid, it is already saturated with moisture and cannot accept any more. So the sweat will not vaporize; it will merely drip down the face and body and exert no cooling effect. In conditions of very high humidity, therefore, sweating becomes ineffective as a means of reducing body temperature.

On a windy day, the process of evaporation has an advantage. The air next to the sweating skin, as soon as it becomes heavily laden with sweat moisture, is blown away, and its place is taken by air that is drier and more receptive to further evaporation.

Clothing is an important factor. It should allow free movement of air over the skin. Trapped pockets of air become saturated with vaporized sweat and prevent further evaporation from that area. Air is a very good insulator and prevents body heat from escaping by conduction or radiation. Examples of clothing that prevent adequate heat loss are the rubberized training suit, or the footballer's uniform, with its plastic helmet and padding, designed to protect against bodily contact injury but not against the ill effects of high heat conditions. Deaths from heatstroke due to the wearing of such apparel are, sad to say, recorded from time to time in the medical literature.

A further condition affecting sweat evaporation has to do with blood volume. When exercising on a hot day, you sweat heavily and lose water from your blood at the rate of 2.5 quarts (2.3 liters) per hour. Unless you replace the sweat loss by drinking fluids, the net result will be a reduction in blood volume. But as long as you keep jogging, your muscles require oxygen and thus your heart is committed to pumping a steady supply of oxygen-laden blood to the scene of action. With the drop in the amount of blood available, however, there is a drop in the amount ejected with each heartbeat. The only way that the heart can now maintain its output of blood is to increase the number of strokes per minute. In other words, the heart rate must go up if the heart is to maintain an adequate blood supply to the exercising muscles.

If you continue to exercise at the same intensity, your maximum heart rate is eventually reached. When that happens, cardiac output cannot keep pace with demand. Actually, you can gain a very slight respite by constricting the blood vessels of the skin, a stratagem that shunts some blood back into the central pool, raising the central blood volume, and once more makes blood available for the heart to pump. Unfortunately, the price you have paid for this temporary postponement of the inevitable is a high one. By diverting blood away from the skin, you have deprived yourself of your major mechanism of heat loss. Thus, the temperature inside your body rapidly begins to climb, and the whole heat-control compensatory system begins to break down. Unless you stop exercising, or unless you have been drinking ample quantities of fluid to replenish your blood volume, you have reached the stage of dehydration.

There are three clinical conditions associated with exercising in the hot weather. Although they may merge imperceptibly and insidiously into one another, to understand the whole mechanism of dehydration let us deal with them as separate entities.

Heat Cramps

Heat cramps occur in highly trained individuals who are working for an hour or more in hot weather. They may come on toward the end of an exercise session or after it, for example, in the shower. They can be extremely severe and may last for many minutes.

Such cramps are thought to be due to a chronic lack or loss of sodium. As I explained earlier, the highly conditioned athlete has a copious sweat production, much greater than the sedentary individual. While the sweat contains less sodium than normal (the body's attempt to conserve its supply), this can be outbalanced by the speed with which sweating occurs, so that eventually there is a tendency to lose sodium. Over the short term, the fluid can be replaced by drinking water, but this does not replace sodium. Ingestion of a dilute salt solution (one teaspoonful of salt to one quart, or 5 milliliters of salt to 1 liter) will relieve the cramps very rapidly.

The average walker or jogger is not likely to be bothered by these heat cramps. They are much more frequent
in the individual who is training for long periods in the
heat. Incidentally, your best sources of salt are ketchup,
bran, fish, nuts, and meat. Do not use salt tablets; they are
far too concentrated a source.

Heat Exhaustion
This condition results from an inadequate replacement of
the water lost in sweat. The early signs are fatigue and
weakness. I cannot emphasize enough that thirst is a very
poor indicator that you need fluid. The mere act of putting
something in the mouth, a pebble, for instance, reduces the
sensation of thirst for about 15 minutes. Laboratory experiments have shown that the introduction of a small
amount of fluid through a tube directly into the stomach
has the same effect—even though the water has not been
absorbed through the stomach wall. So you may take just
a mouthful of cold water, swallow it, no longer feel thirsty,
and carry on exercising for another half an hour before you
feel the need to drink again, yet the amount of fluid taken
is totally inadequate.

With water losses of up to 5% of body weight, the
dehydrated exerciser develops a flushed, hot skin, judgment becomes poor, movement is uncoordinated and
behavior irrational. Other symptoms of heat exhaustion
are light-headedness, a very rapid heart rate, and severe
frontal headaches. Heat exhaustion can occur in varying
degrees of severity and may become chronic during a long
spell of hot-weather training. Drinking adequate amounts
of water before, during, and after training walks or jogs is
just as important as during a football game or a marathon
run. Heat exhaustion can also develop rapidly during
exercise and may progress to heatstroke, the third and
most dangerous manifestation of dehydration.

Heatstroke

Heatstroke is the popular term for hyperpyrexia, that is, body temperature in excess of 108°F (42°C). Again, the cause is lack of water. Its onset can be insidious and rapid. The victims, after demonstrating evidence of extreme heat exhaustion, collapse into a coma, from which they may never recover. Death is frequently due to kidney failure.

The effects of heatstroke on the body are widespread. There is destruction of the specialized cells in the posterior portion of the brain. For this reason, survivors may be left with staggering gait, or speech disorders. Bleeding into the cortex of the brain is responsible for various mental disturbances. The kidneys can be irreparably damaged, making renal dialysis necessary. Hemorrhaging into the heart muscle, and even heart attacks in spite of perfectly normal coronary arteries, have been reported. Clotting of blood in the blood vessels may lead to damage in a whole host of organs. As you can see, an incredible number of deadly pathological changes all stem from simple failure to drink adequately during hot-weather exercise.

How to Avoid Dehydration

Anyone who exercises on a hot day, old or young, male or female, walker, jogger, or runner, is a potential dehydration victim. If you are a fun jogger, never forget that the number of calories burned (and therefore the amount of body heat generated) doesn't depend on the speed you jog, but rather on the distance you cover. For example, whether you jog 3 miles (5 kilometers) in 24 minutes or in 36, you will still burn approximately the same number of calories. Remember that if you are a long-distance walker, the slower the pace, the longer you are exposed to the sun, and so the greater the likelihood of dehydration.

The ratio of your body weight to your surface area (W/SA ratio) is an important factor in your ability to cope with heat. The larger your surface area, the more you can lose heat to the surrounding air. On the other hand, the greater your muscle mass, the more heat you generate when exercising. If you have a high W/SA ratio (short, muscular stature), then you have difficulty coping with hot-weather exercise. You will produce lots of heat, but will be unable to dissipate it rapidly. On the other hand, if you have a low W/SA ratio (tall, slim build), you will have fewer problems during your summer exercise sessions.

The following rules apply equally to middle-aged novice exercisers, joggers, and walkers of all sizes, and highly trained athletes:

1. Allow time for heat acclimatization. The body learns to cope with heat if you give it enough time to adjust. The process takes about seven to ten days, and during this time, the workouts should be low-key to commence with, gradually building up to your usual intensity and duration.

   The benefits of acclimatization were all too apparent during the Desert Storm Campaign, where one of the U.S. military's greatest concerns was the problem of dehydration. Troops from the hotter areas of the country had many fewer problems with heatstroke and related conditions during training than those from colder states.

   When the temperature and/or humidity is high, consult Appendix C for use of the Heat Safety Index.

2. Always prehydrate 10 to 20 minutes or so before exercising on a warm day. Drink about 1 cup (250 milliliters) of fluid, then another 1 cup every 20 minutes or so while working out. Don't wait to feel thirsty before drinking.

3. The best fluid to use is water. It should be comfortably cold (best temperature for absorption is about 40°F (4.4°C), and if you require a flavor you may add a lit-

tle fruit juice according to taste. Minerals such as sodium and potassium aren't really essential; the body can replace them later. However, if you do add sodium, it should be in small amounts of 1 teaspoon (5 milliliters) of salt to 1 gallon (3.8 liters) of water.

4. Some postcoronary exercisers may be taking hydrochlorothiazide medication, a diuretic that is given to treat mild cases of high blood pressure. Diuretics encourage the kidneys to excrete sodium and, therefore, water. Potassium is lost in the urine at the same time, and the prescribing physician often suggests that a patient on such medication increase his or her consumption of potassium-containing foods or, alternatively, prescribes a potassium pill. Obviously, a patient taking diuretics (trade names, Diuril, HydroDiuril, Esiberix) is most susceptible to low blood potassium levels in high-heat training and should be aware of this. Too much or too little potassium in the blood can give rise to various abnormalities of cardiac rhythm. In unexplained cases of palpitations or skipped beats appearing in a healthy exerciser, analysis of a blood sample for potassium concentrations should be carried out.

Other medications that may affect tolerance of heat are beta-blockers. They reduce the rate of sweating and so may predispose to heat stress. Alcohol also acts as a diuretic and so should be avoided before exercise. Furthermore, it impairs judgment and may encourage ill-advised overexertion.

Sugar, usually in the form of glucose, is often added to replacement fluid to provide energy. Actually, there is little to recommend this practice. Glucose solutions that exceed 2.5% strength are too concentrated to be absorbed through the gut wall and therefore lie in the stomach, causing nausea and vomiting. Worse still, to dilute the glucose, water is actually drawn out of the bloodstream and cells of the body into the intestine, thus aggravating the dehydration! If, on the other hand, you prepare a solution containing less than 2.5% glucose, the amount of energy provided is probably too small to be of any value.

The best replacement fluid, then, is still cold water, plus a mild flavoring agent if desired.

5. Clothing should be light, porous, and comfortable. Fishnet vests are most suitable, allowing easy circulation of air and free evaporation of sweat from the skin.

6. Cold water sponging helps, as will putting ice under your hat. If you sponge your legs, be careful not to wet your shoes and socks, otherwise you may develop blisters.

7. Get into the habit of weighing yourself naked before and after each workout. If you have hydrated adequately, you should have lost no more than 3% of your body weight; more than 5%, and you have definitely dehydrated.

8. Finally, when the air temperature and humidity are both extremely high even copious quantities of water will not hold your body temperature down. Slowing your pace, or even walking, will reduce your body's rate of heat generation, but if you start to develop symptoms of excessive body temperature (muscle and abdominal cramps, dizziness, a tendency to stumble), then smarten up and quit exercising. Failure to do so may have very unpleasant consequences.

Do Be Careful in Cold Weather

While indoor exercising has its advocates, I believe that walking and jogging out-of-doors has much to recommend it. Apart from the sheer boredom and discomfort of indoor exercising (when did you last sweat your way round 4 miles [6.5 kilometers] of a "26-laps-to-the-mile" track?), the outdoor exerciser achieves an exhilaration and sense of satisfaction that can be obtained only by physically coping with the natural elements. Besides, if you are going to work out five days a week for the rest of your life, surely the most convenient way to do so is by stepping through your front door and using your own district as a training ground. You fit your exercising into your lifestyle, and you make it part of your daily living.

There are, of course, some hazards associated with exercising in the cold. There is no doubt that the body's reaction to cold puts a stress on the cardiovascular system. When the body temperature falls, it tries to conserve heat by constricting the blood vessels in the skin. This action shunts the warm blood away from the surface and reduces heat loss from conduction, convection, and radiation. The cost of this sudden narrowing of a major portion of the blood vessel system is a rapid rise in the pressure against which the heart is pumping—in other words, a rise in blood pressure. The additional load on the heart brought about by the increase in Rate Pressure Product (HR $\times$ BP) may be sufficient to induce angina in an individual with narrowed coronary arteries.

How is it, though, that tens of thousands of people, from the young to the elderly, can walk, jog, cross-country ski, and skate, with considerable exhilaration and pleasure, despite freezing temperatures? The answer is that the body heat generated by physical activity balances the heat lost to the surrounding air. Skin temperature is therefore maintained at about 92°F (33°C) and a comfortable equilibrium is reached. Cold-induced constriction of skin blood vessels does not occur, and there is no increase in the work load placed upon the heart. However, of the two variables (heat loss and heat production), the ability to generate adequate body heat from exercise may be the most difficult for the person with coronary artery disease. If physical effort is difficult because of angina, heat loss may exceed heat production, and the chain of events just described is set in motion.

In practice, however, cold-weather angina may be avoided in patients with coronary artery disease. Wearing three or four layers of suitable light clothing increases heat-retaining properties without adding to energy expenditure. For instance, an additional energy expenditure of only four or five calories per minute (for example, walking 1 mile in 15 minutes, or 1 kilometer in 9 minutes), can be accomplished in temperatures even as low as 14°F (–10°C) when you are suitably clothed. Those who develop angina in cold weather even when walking very slowly should exercise outdoors only in warmer weather until training results in a drop in Rate Pressure Product and, thus, angina, for a given level of effort. Eventually, they will be able to exercise in colder temperatures.

Some patients who are capable of higher effort levels still suffer angina within a minute or so of beginning their exercise in the cold. The mechanism responsible is probably reflex coronary vasoconstriction. During exercise, as respiratory rate increases, mouth breathing becomes easier. The warming effect of the blood vessels in the mucous membrane of the nose is bypassed, and cold air stimulates the nerve endings at the back of the throat. This in turn leads to spasm of the coronary arteries. Careful indoor warm-up exercise and the use of a woolen scarf covering the mouth may help. In 1968, the Toronto Centre devised a simple, disposable plastic oxygen mask attached to 12 inches (30 centimeters) of flexible tubing extending to beneath the subject's T-shirt to about the level of the chest bone. At a cost of about $10, this easily produced apparatus is highly effective in preventing early-onset cold-induced angina. (It is, incidentally, also effective for patients with emphysema.)

In addition to the possibility of cold-induced angina, we have the problem of snow-covered and icy surfaces, which impose greater energy expenditure and increase the likelihood of injury. Head winds increase chilling effect and air resistance. Rain or wet snow reduces the insulating properties of clothing and allows body heat to "wick out" to the atmosphere. Paradoxically, dehydration can be as much of a problem in the winter as it is in the summer. The evaporative process continues, making excessive fluid loss by sweating possible. Moreover, exposure to cold air strongly suppresses the sense of thirst, and drinking to replace fluid is often ignored.

Fortunately, the body heat generated by fast walking or jogging is usually sufficient to offset loss of heat to the surrounding cold air. Where there is imbalance in favor of heat loss, this can be prevented by wearing suitable clothing.

The purpose of clothing in cold weather is to insulate the surface of the skin from the surrounding environment and prevent heat loss. Clothing traps air and modifies the skin's so-called microclimate. The fabric is less important in this regard than the weave. Layering garments and varying the closeness of the weave or knit allows considerable flexibility in achieving the desired level of heat retention. However, insulating properties may be changed drastically by the action of water or sweat. Tightly woven cotton with little interfiber air-trapping sticks to the body when wet, eliminates large air pockets, and reduces insulation. Wool, on the other hand, retains its insulating properties with its natural oils and greater air-trapping interstices even when wet. In recent years, synthetic fibers have been woven and knit in various ways to develop systems of functional clothing for cold weather activities of all types.

The layer next to the skin should be tightly woven ribbed material that provides some insulation while allowing for evaporation during excessive sweating. The middle layer (loosely woven wool or a fishnet cotton and synthetic mix) should absorb some of this excess sweat but still allow for evaporation. The third layer (a tighter woven wool, wool/cotton combination, or synthetic fiber) should have some degree of stretch to permit variable insulation by opening and closing the weave in the material in response to body movement. A fourth layer is needed only in conditions of high wind and extreme cold. It should protect against wind, rain, and snow, and yet be permeable to body heat. Synthetic materials have performed these functions with considerable success.

If possible, all upper body garments should be zipped or buttoned in such a way that they can be loosened at the neck when the body overheats or closed up if chilling occurs. Dark or colored outer garments tend to conserve body heat; they should be adorned with reflective strip material so as to be visible in the darkness.

The legs rarely require more than two layers. Track suit pants over pantyhose will suffice on even the coldest days. Long underwear is fine, although it tends to restrict knee movement unless it is cut down to shorts length. Socks should be a wool/cotton mixture or a ribbed and channeled, woven synthetic material. Hands, susceptible to cold because they are poorly muscled and used little in jogging, are best protected by wool mittens, which trap more air than gloves. Since considerable body heat is lost through the head, a woolen hat that pulls down over the ears to prevent frostbite is necessary: on very cold days a balaclava, which leaves only the eyes, nose, and mouth exposed, is a good idea. The exposed parts of the face should be protected from chapping and cold sores by applying petroleum jelly. Shoes with waffle soles give greater purchase on ice.

Air temperature is only one of the factors that should be taken into consideration when planning workouts in cold climates. Wind conditions, presence or absence of sunshine, and humidity all affect the body cooling rate.

A 15-mile-an-hour (24-kilometer-an-hour) wind can make a still-air temperature reading of 36°F (2°C) feel like

16°F (–9°C); thus, a wind chill chart should always be consulted on a windy day (see Appendix D).

Is the sun shining or is it overcast? Direct sunshine is worth an additional 13°F (7°C). This can be critical. You may start your walk on a calm day with the sun shining brightly, and if you are using an out-and-back course, by the time you head for home you may find yourself battling a 10-mile-an-hour (16-kilometer-an-hour) wind, with the sun long since disappeared behind the clouds. You are no longer adequately dressed, and things soon become pretty miserable. You can, of course, pick up your pace to generate more body heat. But this may require a level of exertion beyond your capabilities, in which case you will fatigue, lose your body heat even more rapidly or, if you are a postcoronary patient, develop angina and have to slow down again.

Probably the greatest threat to maintaining equilibrium between heat production and heat loss is wet clothing. Whether the cause is driving rain, melting snow, or drenching perspiration, the effect is the same. Evaporation from the wet material will drop your body temperature at an alarming rate. This is one of the most potent causes of hypothermia. With every two degrees Fahrenheit (one degree Celsius) fall below normal, you go through the successive stages of slurred speech, uncoordination of hands and feet, unsteadiness, collapse, and finally coma. Hypothermia is hardly the lot of everyone who goes for a walk or jog on a cold day and gets their clothes wet, but you should take precautions to see that you never put yourself in the position of risking such a tragedy.

Putting all of this together, we can lay down the following guidelines for cold-weather exercising:

1. Wear layers of clothing that are woven to regulate heat loss.

2. Always consult the wind chill chart (see Appendix D) on windy days and use the effective temperature rather than the air temperature as a guideline. If the effective temperature is below 14°F (–10°C), postcoronary exercisers should question the wisdom of exercising out-of-doors.

3. Because the wind and sun conditions can change rapidly, a short out-and-back course should be chosen, the furthest point of which should be no more than a quarter of a mile (half a kilometer) from the starting point. This is particularly important for the less fit.

4. In wet and cold conditions, the clothing layers should include a light cotton and nylon mixture outer garment that will provide two to three hours of protection against moisture.

5. Head winds must be taken into consideration and the pace adjusted downward to maintain the prescribed level of energy expenditure. If one does not reduce pace in the teeth of a head wind, then premature fatigue will inevitably ensue, a slower pace will lead to inadequate heat production, and symptoms from chilling will occur.

By how much should the pace be slowed? Pulse rate during normal workout conditions may be used as a guideline. Alternatively, back off the pace until you are experiencing the same level of breathing rate and leg muscle exertion you usually associate with your customary exercise pace, generally 12 or 13 on the numerical Borg Scale of Perceived Exertion (page 208). This will correlate with the heart rate, blood pressure, and oxygen intake associated with your usual workout, even though, because of difficult or adverse conditions such as head winds or hilly terrain, the speed of the walk/jog is necessarily slower. I find this is true for many of my patients, but it does cause problems in those "deniers" who consistently overestimate their prowess. It can also be a dangerous rule of thumb for patients who develop increased skipped beats with exercise and who can detect them only by pulse taking.

6. Frostbite is unusual in the walker/jogger, but can occur in poorly protected hands, ears, and faces exposed to temperatures below 30°F (−1°C). Failure to take wind chill into account is usually the cause.

Since its inception, a high percentage of patients on the Toronto program have walked and jogged out-of-doors throughout the winter on all but the severest days without ill effects. They are the finest testimonial to our approach. The trouble is, by the time winter has come to an end, they have to start acclimatizing to the heat again. Such is life!

Don't Do Heavy Isometric Exercises

A maximum isometric muscle contraction is one in which the muscle contracts with full force but without shortening. For example, normally, when the biceps muscle in your upper arm contracts, your elbow bends. If you contract the muscle while at the same time holding the elbow joint rigid, you have achieved an isometric contraction of your biceps. Examples of isometric effort in everyday life are straining to raise a jammed window, trying to lift a too-heavy suitcase, or attempting to push a snow-bound automobile. This type of muscle action, as opposed to the "isotonic" movement in which the joint is allowed to move and the muscle to shorten, causes a sharp rise in the diastolic blood pressure and a marked increase in the pressures within the chambers of the heart. If the heart wall is scarred from a previous heart attack, and if the coronary blood circulation is impaired as a result of atherosclerosis, the results of such pressure increases can be dangerous.

An example of the adverse cardiovascular effects of an

isometric effort is found in Lord Moran's book on Sir Winston Churchill:

> *Washington, December 17. "I am glad you have come,"*
> *Churchill began. He was in bed and looked worried. "It*
> *was hot last night, and I got up to open the window. It*
> *was very stiff. I had to use considerable force and I*
> *noticed all at once I was short of breath. I had a dull pain*
> *over my heart. It went down my left arm. It did not last*
> *very long, but it has never happened before. What is it?*
> *Is my heart all right? I thought of sending for you, but it*
> *passed off."*

Sir Winston was an astute observer of symptoms. He was describing typical angina pectoris as the result of an excessive load on his heart and coronary vasculature.

An additional problem with all isometric exercises is that the uninitiated tend to hold their breath while carrying them out. While this may seem to enhance performance, it introduces another element of danger for the person with heart problems. A not uncommon sight in any gymnasium is an exerciser slowly going blue in the face as he attempts to strain himself to the limit. By holding his breath, he has closed off his windpipe, and in the course of his exercise is forcing the air into his lungs against the closed valve. This state of affairs is referred to in physiological circles as the Valsalva maneuver. Its effect, like that of the isometric muscle contraction, is to throw a heavy burden on a heart already severely taxed by the particular exercise that is being carried out. So remember—never hold your breath when straining to push or lift an excessive load.

Do Take Care When Shoveling Snow
The incidence of fatal heart attack and sudden cardiac death in any large city inevitably mounts in the three or

four days after a heavy snowstorm. These deaths are almost entirely the result of snow shovelling, which has particularly adverse effects on the elderly and those with coronary artery disease. The activity has all the components necessary to put the cardiovascular system in jeopardy. It is not only a very intense form of exercise, equivalent to running a mile (1.6 kilometers) at anywhere between 7 and 12 minutes (depending on whether you are moving heavy wet or dry light snow); it is also usually performed under unfavorable conditions of extreme cold. Add to that the most dangerous element of all—the repeated isometric arm contractions, customarily accompanied by the Valsalva maneuver, and you have set the stage for potential disaster.

If you have to move snow, do it as follows. Dress for the cold in the manner advised under the section on "Cold Weather Exercise" earlier in this chapter, and always warm up for four or five minutes before starting. Push the snow with a scoop rather than lifting it with a shovel; this action allows your legs to do the work isotonically rather than your arms isometrically. Take a rest every three minutes or so and don't let yourself get out of breath. If you suffer from angina, or have severe coronary artery disease, give the chore to someone else!

Does this mean that you must be in constant fear of holding your breath or inadvertently carrying out an isometric muscle contraction? Of course not. As a matter of fact, the more endurance fitness you develop, the stronger your heart, and the more it will be able to resist such stresses and strains.

Do Beware of Saunas and Steam Baths
Postcoronary patients have been found to develop electrocardiographic evidence of myocardial ischemia while in the sauna; these changes took the form of ST segment depression and frequent ectopic beats. They did not occur

to anything like the same extent when these same subjects exercised to a heart rate level equivalent to that attained in the sauna. The reason for this is that excessive heat, like emotional stress, releases large quantities of noradrenaline and adrenaline into the bloodstream, which may have adverse effects on the myocardium. Potentially dangerous falls in blood pressure levels have been reported as a result of dilation of skin vessels (especially when the subject is in the sitting position) with resultant decrease in coronary blood flow.

Steam baths, whirlpools, and hot tubs utilize moist heat, which is the least well tolerated by the body, since it prevents loss of heat by evaporation, or sweating, and permits the body temperature to rise more quickly to sometimes dangerous levels. Saunas, on the other hand, because they use dry heat, permit sweating, but are often very hot, 170°F (77°C), or more. The excessive sweating can cause dehydration. The loss of water from the blood makes the blood thicker and more likely to clot inside an atherosclerotic coronary, and possibly cause a heart attack.

If you use the sauna, drink plenty of water to replace that lost in the sweat. Choose a cooler type of bath, or limit the stay in higher temperatures to five minutes. Do not use the steam bath to "sweat out" symptoms that might well be the early warning of coronary artery disease (for example, "muscular" chest pain, excessive fatigue, or "bursitis" in the shoulder). Above all, do not, out of a false sense of pride, attempt to "tough it out" if you feel yourself getting dizzy, breathless, or developing an unpleasant thumping of your heart.

Don't Exercise When Pollution Levels Are High

What are the common air pollutants? What effect do they have on us? The answer to the first question depends on the area in which you live. In Los Angeles, for instance, the pollutants are composed largely of compounds that arise from the chemical interaction between sunlight and the various combustible products of automobile fumes. In other cities, we may be dealing predominantly with carbon monoxide, sulphur dioxide, or a number of airborne chemicals in particulate form.

Carbon monoxide is a major component of cigarette smoke, and we have already described how it occupies the red cells of the blood, displacing the vital oxygen being carried to the body's cells. Inhaled even in minute quantities by the exerciser, it could reduce the efficiency of their oxygen transport system and turn an easy workout into a relatively tough one. Inhaling enough carbon monoxide to affect about 20% of the hemoglobin, the oxygen-carrying protein in the blood, will lead to headache behind and over the eyes, breathlessness, muscular weakness, and dizziness. When about 40% of the available hemoglobin is saturated with carbon monoxide, there is a feeling of nausea, severe headache, and breathlessness on exertion, together with dimming and blurring of vision; judgment becomes impaired and the individual becomes belligerent; there is lack of coordination, stumbling, and possibly even collapse. Some studies have shown that patients with coronary heart disease can develop angina or electrocardiographic evidence of myocardial ischemic changes with carbon monoxide levels as low as 3% to 5%. Thus, since the major source of carbon monoxide is from automobile exhaust fumes, you should avoid walking or jogging close to heavily traveled main streets or highways. Exhaust smoke, however, disperses slowly, so if your jogging route is 40 to 60 feet (12 to 18 meters) or more away from the edge of a busy highway, you should reduce the risk; better still, try to find a route through a park, green belt, or a relatively smog-free suburb.

Ozone is a key component in the smog that results from the action of sunlight on fuel-oil hydrocarbons and nitrogen dioxide. It has been found in aircraft cabins at altitudes above 30,000 feet, and also in association with various welding devices. In recent years, a good deal of work has been carried out on the effect of ozone on the human body, and while much is still to be learned, we do have some indications that in high concentrations (greater than 0.15 parts per million of air), it can have some toxic effect. Its major target is the respiratory organs, where it can cause breathlessness, chest pain, and coughing. In addition to the respiratory symptoms, high ozone levels can cause headaches and reduce one's ability to concentrate. The heart rate may decrease, and this can give rise to increases in blood carbon dioxide. At ozone levels in excess of 0.2 parts per million, there may be a considerable decrease in central visual acuity and ability to see in the dark. Some coaches have reported that when the ozone levels are high, athletic performance is adversely affected.

A few cities now operate an ozone alert when the level reaches more than 0.15 parts per million, which warns susceptible individuals to reduce physical exertion. When the level becomes in excess of 0.2 parts per million, even healthy persons should limit their outdoor exercise. It is possible, however, to defeat the ozone problem if you remember one or two basic principles. In the first place, keep in mind that on a sunny, humid day the maximal ozone levels occur between 11:00 a.m. and 6:00 p.m., and the lowest levels occur in the early morning. Therefore, if you wish to be on the safe side, exercise early in the morning or late at night. Older individuals (and that means us) are more susceptible to the effects of ozone than young people. Don't forget that the hotter it gets, the more ozone is produced. Secondly, if you have a chest infection, you are obviously more susceptible. Interestingly, the ingestion of vitamin C would appear to substantially reduce the effect of ozone on the lungs. Finally (and this must be a consolation to Los Angeleans), the more exposure you

have to ozone, the more likely you are to develop a tolerance toward it. At least you are less likely to be overcome
by the more acute and unpleasant symptoms.

There is no doubt that running in the city on a hot,
humid, muggy day when the traffic is heavy and the
industrial pall is hanging close to the ground can be
uncomfortable and sometimes downright unpleasant.
Nevertheless, if you follow these simple guidelines you
should not come to any harm, and the benefits of exercising will far outweigh any minor and transitory discom-
forts brought about by breathing polluted air.

Don't Exercise with a Fever
A number of viral-type infections can involve the heart
muscle. The effect may be transitory, lasting only a matter
of days or weeks. They may pass unnoticed by the patient
and leave no permanent damage. However, strenuous
physical activity should be avoided during this time.
Although severe viral myocarditis is relatively rare, mild
forms of the condition may exist much more frequently
than we suspect. Since a visit to the cardiologist is hardly
justified every time you develop a fever, be safe rather
than sorry: don't exercise if you are suffering from any flu-
like illness. To be further on the safe side, you should not
work out until 72 hours after your temperature has
returned to normal.

Don't Abuse Alcohol
Excessive alcohol intake can contribute to obesity and
hypertension. Alcohol is a major health problem in many
countries today. On the other hand, a number of studies
have suggested that light to moderate drinking is associated with a lower incidence of heart attacks than in non-
drinking or heavy drinking. The reason seems to be that
alcohol in moderation raises HDL-cholesterol and prevents excessive blood clotting. The upper limit of mod-

erate drinking is defined as being no more than two drinks a day.

Having said that, I should emphasize that it is very easy to exceed the "moderate" level. In the patient with coronary disease, alcohol can also depress heart function. The amount of alcohol needed to cause this adverse effect in heart patients is quite small: in one study, just 2 ounces (60 milliliters) of whisky. The heart muscle cells may also suffer permanent damage from prolonged and excessive alcohol consumption. Another practical consideration is body weight. Alcoholic beverages are high in caloric value, so you can scarcely expect to lose weight on a diet of cottage cheese, lettuce, and beer!

For all of the above reasons, consider carefully whether or not to consume alcohol. If you have serious cardiac problems, you are better off abstaining. Chances are, however, that if you are capable of exercising, you are capable of drinking, but in moderation.

Just as you shouldn't drink and drive, so you should never drink before jogging, especially if you suffer from heart disease. Not only is your heart less likely to be able to cope with the additional stress, but your judgment of pace and distance is probably impaired, as is your ability to count your pulse and interpret such warning signs as angina or light-headedness. If you do drink, then do so in moderation, and *after* your workout.

Do Check the Physical Conditions

Don't underestimate the effect of running into a head wind. It has been shown that an athlete weighing 134 pounds (61 kilograms) and running at a 6-minute-mile (3.75-minute-kilometer) pace on a still day will expend approximately 6% more oxygen if he runs at the same pace but into a light, 10 mph (16 kmph) head wind. To put it another way, he will have to put out the effort of a sub-five-minute-mile (sub-three-minute-kilometer) pace! At

40 mph (64 kmph), head wind increases the oxygen cost by over 40%. When you are talking oxygen increments of that order, you may be getting into a situation that is beyond your maximal oxygen intake. The trick is to back off if you notice yourself getting unusually breathless and tired on a windy day. Allowing for the wind resistance, the slower time will be giving you the same training effect anyway.

The best surface to run on is a smooth one. The hardness or softness doesn't really matter; your shoes should take care of that factor. An uneven surface considerably increases the effort of running, driving up your oxygen intake and heart rate accordingly, and sometimes giving rise to anginal pain that would otherwise not occur. Some athletes feel that it is easier to run on a grass surface and will seek one out if they are trying to nurse a leg injury. In my experience, this only makes matters worse, since beneath the deceptive green covering, the underlying ground is often rutted and uneven, making each stride a hazard and increasing the stress on tendons and ligaments. If possible, then, do your training on the road or on a track with a good surface.

13. Facts and Fallacies

One of the features of the Toronto program is the question-and-answer sessions which follow the formal lectures and precede the exercise workouts. The following topics are those most commonly covered in these informal chats. I hope they will clarify a few of your problems and correct some of the half-truths, fallacies, and prejudices with which the exercising heart patient is surrounded.

Sexual Activity after a Heart Attack

Half our postcoronary patients reported a reduction in sexual activity after their heart attack. The main reason given was a fall-off in desire. A smaller number said that they were frightened of suffering another heart attack during intercourse, and a few actually reported adverse symptoms such as palpitations or angina pectoris during the sexual act.

The individual who becomes apathetic toward sex after the attack frequently shows high levels of depression and anxiety. The reluctance to seek full satisfaction in sexual relations is perfectly understandable under these circumstances. As confidence returns (and this often occurs with increasing physical fitness), the situation usually rights itself.

But what of the individual who is frightened of sexual intercourse because of its possible ill effects on the heart? Is there any justification for these fears? Should special precautions be observed during the sex act, and if so, what should they be? How long should one wait after the heart attack before resuming a normal sexual relationship?

The answers to these questions may have been provided by your cardiologist, but I find that many of the patients referred for rehabilitation have been given little guidance in this area. The reason is not hard to find. Minimal research has been carried out into the effects of coitus on the damaged heart, and medical literature contains little on the subject.

The sex act results in cardiovascular responses very similar to those induced by exercise. There is a rise in heart rate and blood pressure, as well as an increase in the rate of breathing. However, in terms of cardiac work, the cost of intercourse is modest, with increases in heart rate about the same as that observed in climbing a few flights of stairs or walking briskly around the block. As a matter of fact, much higher heart rates may occur during angry discussions at work! ECG monitoring of 14 subjects during the sexual act showed that a small number developed changes compatible with cardiac ischemia (ST segment depression and ectopic beats), but these particular individuals experienced similar adverse signs during their usual occupational activities; in other words, coitus did not have a disproportionately higher stress effect.

The vast majority of postcoronary patients can safely indulge in marital sexual activity without fear of excessive cardiovascular strain. Here we refer to middle-aged individuals who have been married for a number of years. There are grounds for believing that intercourse with a younger or less familiar partner may lead to more profound physiological changes, with much higher increments of heart rate and blood pressure and therefore greater cardiac stress. Extramarital intercourse may well provide these ingredients, and since it may also be accompanied by a bout of excessive food and alcohol intake, might well be dangerous. It is probably in these circumstances that the occasional coitus death occurs—a death dramatic enough to become more colorful in the retelling, and so needlessly frighten the more conservative members of society!

Are there precautions to be taken after a heart attack? Sufficient time should be allowed after the attack before indulging in intercourse. Wait three to four weeks after the attack, or until you can go for a brisk walk or climb two flights of stairs without difficulty. If you suffer from angina during coitus, then try taking glyceryl trinitrate before commencing the act. Symptoms such as angina or ectopic beats may be relieved by changing your position. Supporting your body weight on your arms amounts to isometric exercise and, as previously noted, will lead to a disproportionate increase in blood pressure and cardiac work load. The effect is enhanced if the duration of the act is prolonged. Therefore, if you are bothered by symptoms, try the side-by-side position or have your partner take the top position.

Depression Following Heart Attack
Our own studies, as well as the work of others, have shown that many heart attack survivors pass through a stage of depression following their attack. This is perfectly understandable. After all, for most it is the first time that they have been faced with their own mortality—and in a very dramatic manner. This type of depression is known as *reactive* depression. It is an emotional response to an adverse event. When that event is as serious as a heart attack, it is almost to be expected. Incidentally, reactive depression is a far cry from *endogenous* depression, which is completely out of proportion and often bears no relationship to external cir-

cumstances. This type of depression can be very disabling and requires professional help. Most of our reactively depressed patients pass out of this phase spontaneously in a matter of months. Others may take more time.

The depressed heart patient lacks confidence, shows less initiative at home and work, is reluctant to make important decisions, and constantly procrastinates, hoping that time will solve the problem. At home, more and more responsibility is left to the spouse. This change was so marked in one patient that his wife, before leaving for a holiday, wrote him a note in which she adjured him to pull himself together and revert to the strong-minded man she had married, who had consistently called the shots for both of them.

There is little doubt that great benefit can be derived from an exercise rehabilitation program. Fitness improves the quality of life and brings with it enhanced self-confidence and improvement in morale. Our depressed patients have gained considerably from the exercise program. However, we have learned to take a slightly different approach with our depressed as opposed to our nondepressed patients. Initially, they tend to be overly protective, frightened of exertion, doubtful of the program's value, pessimistic about their own chances of improvement, and inclined to do less than the prescription calls for. They allow any number of trivial excuses to deflect them from the exercise session, frequently complain of leg muscle stiffness, or vague discomfort in the chest, and constantly seem to be searching for an excuse to drop out. They need encouragement, reassurance, and a high degree of persuasion to ensure that they keep on exercising at a suitable level. They are helped by observing the success of other postcoronary joggers who are obviously doing so well. If they can just stay with the program long enough to start feeling the benefits of fitness, they are well on the road to recovery.

Denial after the Heart Attack

This is yet another response and one that requires a different approach. These individuals have no sense of insecurity; psychological testing reveals that they have abundant self-confidence. Ambitious, driving, and overcompetitive, they deny adverse symptoms, and even sometimes that they have suffered a heart attack. They are obsessive in their adherence to their exercise workouts. They are constantly matching their performances with those of others and setting themselves harder and harder goals. They are inclined to exceed their exercise prescription and have to be observed carefully in order to see that they do not do too much or ignore the indications for a reduction in training intensity.

Do you recognize yourself as belonging to either of these two groups? If so, consider how your attitude affects your approach to exercise—and to your life in general. Knowledge is power. Knowledge of oneself is even more powerful.

Exercise-related Deaths

Death during or shortly after a bout of exercise is a rare event. It is also a dramatic event and inevitably draws attention, particularly if the victim is a high-profile member of the community. The death of a famous athlete is greeted with considerable alarm, and understandably so. Examples are 28-year-old Sergei Grinkov, the two-time Olympic gold medalist ice skater who died during a training session, Hank Gathers, the basketball star, and Jim Fixx, the author of the best-seller, *The Art of Running*, who died during an early morning 6-mile (10-kilometer) jog. By focusing attention on the advantages and disadvantages of exercise, the wide publicity given to these individuals' deaths served a valuable purpose. On the other hand, if it led people to believe that taking up exercise in order to become physically fit was a life-threatening procedure, it did a great disservice. Regular physical exercise is clearly an important part of a strategy for the prevention of coronary heart disease, and one of the manifestations of that disease is sudden death. How can these facts be reconciled with the reports one sometimes hears of sudden heart-related deaths that occur when the person is exercising?

Let us put the topic in perspective. In the United States, one in every four people under the age of 50 years who dies of natural causes dies suddenly. The majority of these are due to diseases of the heart or blood vessels, and in those 30 years or older, practically all are due to coronary atherosclerosis. In most cases, the presence of coronary disease had already been diagnosed and the subject was aware of it, but in others there were no prior symptoms and the victim was apparently healthy. The latter cases are labeled medically as "sudden cardiac deaths" (SCDs).

SCD is so common these days that autopsy findings are of medical interest only if they reveal a non-cardiac cause. Furthermore, sudden death in patients with known coronary disease is so taken for granted that autopsy is rarely carried out. At times this can lead to false assumptions. An example is a 68-year-old coronary patient of mine who collapsed and died in the bathroom while getting ready to go out for his morning jog. It was presumed that he died as a result of his coronary disease. However, in life he had requested that autopsy be carried out if he died suddenly. The autopsy revealed that he had died from a very rare inflammatory disease of the heart muscle, sarcoidosis, which had nothing to do with his coronary atherosclerosis, and could have caused his death at any time. Had it happened a short time later, while he was exercising, it would have been labeled an exercise death.

Because of the current worldwide interest in exercise for its health benefits, and the reports from time to time of exercise deaths, public health physicians, cardiology researchers, and statisticians have investigated the problem in some detail.

In a study carried out in Rhode Island, with a population of approximately 1 million, there were 81 exercise-related deaths over the period 1975 to 1982. At first this may seem a lot, but as Dr. William Castelli of Framingham has been heard to say on more than one occasion, in his usual laconic manner, "Sure, that's the numerator but where is the denominator?" By that he means where is the figure showing the number of exercisers overall in Rhode Island, and how often and for how long do they exercise? Without this information, it is hard to put the figure of 81 deaths into perspective.

One of the most informative studies was carried out by Dr. David Siscovik from the University of North Carolina, in association with the Department of Epidemiology, University of Washington. It looked at the incidence of SCD in King County, Washington, which has a population of 1¼ million.

Siscovik was able to show that moderate and high-level habitual exercisers had a baseline death rate from coronary heart disease half that of the sedentary or those with low-level physical activity patterns. In other words, they had a significantly lower risk of coronary death, sudden or otherwise, over any given 24-hour period. However, they did increase their risk of SCD fivefold when they undertook a bout of vigorous physical exercise. Compare that with the sedentary individuals, who increased their risk fifty-six-fold if they exercised vigorously, or encountered an unexpected bout of intense physical activity. On all counts, then, those who were fit came out ahead of the game.

Dr. Murray Mittleman and colleagues investigated the circumstances in the 26-hour period leading up to a heart attack in a large group of patients. Some 4% reported a bout of heavy exertion within an hour before the start of the attack. The activities included shovelling snow, speed walking, jogging, and heavy gardening. All activities were accompanied by breathlessness and sweating, further proof that they were vigorous. For the group as a whole, vigorous exertion increased the risk of SCD five times. However, for the sedentary it increased it one hundred times. The risk fell significantly with training frequency. For those who trained once to twice a week, the relative risk was 20; at three to four times a week, the relative risk was 9; and at five times or more, the relative risk was 2. These findings complement and emphasize those of Siscovik.

People with normal hearts, for all practical purposes, do not suffer exercise SCD. Reports to the contrary are so rare, and so open to question, that they need not concern us here. In the under-30-year-olds, the causes are usually congenital malformation of the coronary vessels of the heart valves, myocarditis or inflammation of the heart muscle, or hypertrophic cardiomyopathy, a disease that enlarges the muscle fibers of the heart and thickens its walls (and which, incidentally, caused the death of Hank Gathers). Sergei Grinkov was an exception. Autopsy revealed that he had suffered a major heart attack a few hours before going on the ice to train. There was, however, a strong hereditary trait, his father dying at the age of 52.

In the over-30-year-olds, rare as exercise SCD is, we know that it is almost always associated with the presence of coronary heart disease, recognized or otherwise. This was the case with Jim Fixx. In such individuals, vigorous exercise can act as a trigger in three ways. It can precipitate the rupture of a thinly capped atherosclerotic plaque which is bulging with liquid fat. In addition, it can cause the dysfunctional coronary endothelium, which has been damaged by atherosclerosis, to constrict rather than dilate in response to an increased blood flow, thus starving the heart muscle of blood at the very time when it is in need of more. Finally, it can increase blood clotting by activating blood platelets and fibrinogen.

How do we interpret all of this information? Well, there is no doubt that if you never exercise, you will never die exercising. On the other hand, no one can avoid occasions when a bout of vigorous exertion is unavoidable. If you are sedentary, we have seen that such an episode increases your relative risk of SCD a hundredfold. Regular exercisers, on the other hand, while being at a slightly higher risk during a vigorous training session, have a much lower overall risk. In the big picture, the absolute risk of exercise-triggered SCD is very small. Nevertheless it is higher in those exercisers who have coronary heart disease, and is more likely in those middle-aged, coronary-prone, sedentary individuals who exercise rarely, and when they do, at an unaccustomed and high level of intensity. These are the weekend athletes, who are inactive all winter, and then play a hard game of tennis on that first good weekend of summer.

If you are a middle-aged casual exerciser, beginner or otherwise, you should not engage in vigorous games such as squash, or indeed any competitive sport, unless you are fit to do so. You can check your fitness level by having a formal fitness test at your local "Y," local health club, or better still, in your physician's office. If this is not possible, then you can carry out the fitness step test outlined in this book, or refer to the cardiovascular fitness tables in the appendices.

Formal cardiac rehabilitation programs have an excellent safety record. However, caution is imperative, and all of these patients have the advantage of undergoing an exercise test, with electrocardiographic monitoring during exercise sessions when indicated, and a medically prescribed, carefully supervised regime. They are taught to recognize and report dangerous symptoms and have a set of rules to follow that reduce their risk of exercise SCD. For those not on such a program, however, the points covered in Chapter 9 should be carefully considered.

The problems of exercising in the heat have been discussed elsewhere but one cannot overemphasize the dangers. Deaths during exercise in high temperatures have been ascribed to heart attacks, and yet on more than one occasion autopsies have failed to reveal any evidence of coronary atherosclerosis. It is not unreasonable to assume that such deaths have been due to dehydration, alteration in blood electrolytes, and perhaps even coronary spasm. No one is immune to all the consequences of dehydration, but middle-aged individuals with latent coronary artery disease are more susceptible.

Another important factor to take into consideration is that of personality. The driving, ambitious individual, once introduced to an exercise program, is usually overeager to excel. If you are one of these, then you will be well-advised to control your tendency toward aggression and competitiveness; it is easy for you to become compulsive and, when business pressures mount, try to complete your workout in a shorter and shorter time. Even worse, you may deny cardiac symptoms in order to keep up your exercise program and still handle heavy business and social commitments. The inherent danger in this attitude is that it always causes a delay before symptoms are brought to the attention of the physician. *Warning signs such as excessive fatigue, tiredness, and especially altered anginal-type chest pain on exercise should be taken very seriously. They are indications that the training must be immediately suspended, pending a detailed re-examination of your cardiovascular status.*

I have evolved five exercise rules that apply particularly to these highly competitive, "deadline" personalities:

- Train regularly, avoiding excessive peaks of activity.
- Avoid intensive competition.
- Adhere to the prescribed limits.

• Report all "cardiac-type" symptoms such as exercise-related chest pain, arm pain, excessive palpitations, dizziness, "blackouts," or undue breathlessness—even if they appear for the first time after years of steady symptom-free training.

To sum up, exercise-induced deaths are very rare, but they do occur and are more likely in the non-conditioned coronary-prone individual, with and without previous evidence of coronary heart disease. Nevertheless, the fact that the recent worldwide explosion in all forms of exercise has not been accompanied by an immediate and proportionate increase in exercise SCD attests in the most dramatic and convincing way possible to the inherent safety of sensible, moderate physical training programs.

Participation in Other Sporting Activities
When can I play tennis? What about golf? Is badminton okay? How about swimming? These and other similar questions are asked constantly by postcoronary patients who are on the exercise program. We try to answer each one individually, taking into account the patient's state of training, age, severity of heart attack, and presence or absence of symptoms. If you are working out in accordance with the training tables in this book, you can use your achievement of the various levels as a rough guide to your ability to participate safely in a number of recreational physical activities (see Appendix E).

Although some of these recreational physical activities may be more enjoyable than jogging, they are harder to quantify in terms of energy expenditure and cardiac work. If you are good at a game, then you will perform it with greater skill, or to put it physiologically, with a higher degree of mechanical efficiency. Thus, your oxygen intake will be lower throughout the game than if you were a less proficient player. A poor swimmer will expend more effort thrashing across the pool than his or her accomplished counterpart in an apparently lazy workout covering many lengths. The squash player with 20 years' experience will finish a game hardly perspiring, while his or her sweating novice opponent may have just had the match of his life.

Other variables in recreational sports include difficulty in pacing oneself, the effect of emotion and excitement, as well as extraneous factors peculiar to the game itself—as for example, the isometric component involved in gripping the ski-tow bar, or the late nights (and possibly the hip-flask conviviality) associated with club curling.

Air Travel

Nowadays, whether for business or vacation, most of us have to fly at some time or another. Can flying pose any special threat for the individual with coronary artery disease? Generally speaking, the answer is no. However, certain considerations have to be taken into account.

Jet planes usually cruise at altitudes of between 30,000 and 40,000 feet (9,144 to 12,192 meters). At these heights, the atmosphere is so rarefied that, were it not for the pressurized cabin, passengers and crew would rapidly expire from a lack of oxygen. Pressurization creates a cabin "altitude" between 5,000 and 7,000 feet (1,524 to 2,134 meters). In effect, the majority of trips are made at cabin altitudes between that equivalent to Denver, Colorado (5,000 feet or 1,524 meters), and Mexico City (7,523 feet or 2,293 meters). This is not a serious problem, since our blood's ability to absorb and transport oxygen through the circulatory system isn't materially hindered until we are exposed to altitudes of 10,000 feet (3,048 meters) and above.

However, individuals with chest disease, such as chronic bronchitis or emphysema, may have difficulty getting sufficient oxygen at lower atmospheric pressures than 10,000 feet (3,048 meters). Obviously, any patient who is breathless at rest, or on minimal exertion, will fly only after very careful medical assessment. As for those with coronary artery disease, the ability to climb two flights of stairs easily or walk 100 yards (91 meters) briskly without breathlessness should ensure a problem-free flight.

How long after a heart attack should one wait before flying? Published reports indicate that fewer problems occur in those whose heart attack has happened two to six months before the flight than in those who fly less than eight weeks after their attack. Those in whom the attack was accompanied by complications, or in whom there was a history of more than one previous attack, also have a higher occurrence of in-flight problems. It would seem wise, then, to defer flying for at least two months. However, if you must travel earlier, then you should check with the airline, all of which have slightly different regulations but will require a physician's letter, and will also leave the final decision to their medical officer.

Actually, in my experience, patients have suffered more episodes of angina on the ground than in the air, particularly as a result of the strain and frustrations of crowded airports, flight delays, customs and immigration inspections, and lengthy waits at baggage conveyors.

Apart from the matter of cabin altitude, there are other aspects of air travel that are probably more important. Alcohol and cigarette smoke intensify the ill effects of low blood oxygen, and so are best avoided, or at least reduced, during long flights. Since the atmosphere in the cabin is dry and rarefied, dehydration can be a problem. Remember, then, to drink plenty of non-alcoholic fluids. Another point to note is that gas expands at altitude. That includes the gas in your stomach. Therefore, on a long flight wear loose clothing, and don't consume too many carbonated drinks, or you'll bloat up like a balloon. Take a walk up and down the cabin every half hour or so to keep the circulation flowing and to avoid blood "pooling" in the lower limbs. If this is not possible, straighten your knees and ankles and clench the thigh and calf muscles from time to time. Finally, and most importantly, always carry three days' supply of your medication on your person or in your cabin luggage. If you pack it in checked luggage, you will sooner or later face the problem of lost bags and, at best, the inconvenience of having to find a local physician to prescribe replacements.

14. Family Matters

This chapter is for husbands, wives, and other relatives of heart patients, and in some ways it is probably one of the most important in the entire book. Why so? Because a change in lifestyle in a partnership means a change for both parties. I will go further. Only with the complete cooperation and understanding of the spouse can the heart attack patient hope to adhere to this or any other cardiac rehabilitation program.

In the Hospital
The problems start immediately with the diagnosis of the heart attack. Nearly half the spouses we interviewed reported being numbed, or in a state of shock on hearing the news. Like the victims, they echo the phrase, "This can't be happening." This sense of unreality is quickly shattered, however, by the day-to-day problems that arise. Most difficult perhaps are the visits to the hospital, which have to be fitted in between the usual daily duties, whether holding down a job, looking after the family, or, more commonly these days, both.

How should you behave during these hospital visits? Above all, your attitude should express confident anticipation of an excellent recovery. In the vast majority of cases, that will be the outcome. Only if the doctors and nurses caution against any optimism should you adopt a sober, realistic approach. Even then, remember that doctors, like weather forecasters, are never right 100% of the time. So feel free to be optimistic and to discuss plans for what you both will do after leaving the hospital. Something good to look forward to is probably the best of all medicines. In the early days in hospital, however, and immediately after coming out of critical care, fatigue is a common symptom. Don't overstay your welcome.

At Home
For the first few weeks after discharge, the patient may be overly dependent and even childlike in attitude. Don't encourage this dependency or be too fearful. As one wife said, "I am scared stiff that I will lose my temper, raise my voice, criticize or do anything that will make him ill again."

A feature of the Toronto program is an evening with the spouses of newly referred patients. It provides an occasion to meet with the staff, and allows us the opportunity to explain the nature of heart disease, its probable causes, and the role that exercise and risk reduction play in prevention. After the talk, the questions start. With audiences of about one hundred assembled, you can imagine that the queries are many and varied. Here are some of the questions most often asked by the concerned partner.

How Can I Overcome Despondency?
It is now accepted that rehabilitation should start as soon as the patient gets out of the coronary care unit and returns to the general ward. For the moment, the patient is glad just to be alive, but as the days pass, that feeling of relief is replaced by one of despondency. The mind is plagued by doubts and uncertainties, all revolving around the ability to do all the things that were part and

parcel of everyday life before the attack. As one patient said to me, "I desperately wanted to get out of the hospital, and yet I was scared to go home. Things I had always taken for granted now became a first. The first time you walk up the stairs, or mow the grass, or clean out the basement, or go back to work, it's the same feeling—will you make it? It's as if you're trying to pick up the pieces of your life again, and never being sure if they'll fit together properly this time."

A good postcoronary rehabilitation program helps to overcome much of this fear. No program, however, can help as much as a well-informed spouse. Take a positive approach right from hospital discharge. Don't avoid discussing the future. The majority of heart attack patients return to their previous lives. If your spouse's is the exceptional case, it still does no harm to discuss alternatives. To make small talk and steer away from a topic as important as future work plans is a great mistake; to the depressed patient, it can only mean one thing—there is no future to discuss.

Avoid being oversolicitous. Exercise sensible precautions, but don't fuss. No doubt certain physical activities are slightly more risky, but then driving an automobile isn't exactly 100% safe these days, and no one can live life completely immune from risk. Besides, until recently, the tendency has been to exaggerate the dangers of physical effort for heart attack patients. We now know that many of the things that they want to do are perfectly safe. Your doctor, or the rehabilitation team, should be able to advise you if there are any important physical restrictions.

In the first few months after the attack, your spouse may be reluctant to make decisions. This is perfectly natural and is just another manifestation of the depressed mood. Eventually, the situation rights itself. Be patient, and whatever you do, don't get into the habit of making all the decisions in the home. If you do, you may well find yourself stuck with the role of decision-maker permanently. Every so often, give your partner the opportunity to regain the initiative.

How Should I React to Symptoms?

Symptom-claiming is not unusual in the early days following the attack. It is an expression of insecurity and represents a need for reassurance. This phase may last a matter of months only, but it can be a real trial for the spouse who never becomes quite accustomed to a succession of frightening complaints of chest pain, numbness in hands, dizziness, and so on. It is difficult not to push the panic button and call the physician on every occasion.

There are, however, some guidelines for action. Severe chest pain (or pain similar to that which accompanied the first attack) that lasts for more than 20 minutes, is not relieved by taking nitroglycerine, lying down or resting, and is accompanied by sweating, pallor, nausea, or vomiting indicates the need for speedy medical assistance. If you can't get the physician, arrange immediate transportation to the emergency department.

There are other indications of impending trouble that, although less dramatic than chest pain, should nevertheless be heeded. Foremost among these is excessive fatigue. Tiredness that is not relieved by a good night's rest should be considered suspect in the recent postcoronary patient, and a search should be made for the cause. A heavy work load or an overcrowded social itinerary is usually the culprit, and steps should be taken immediately to adopt a more sensible and relaxed routine. Frequently, the spouse is the first to recognize the onset of the cantankerous, irritable manner that was so typical of the first attack. Both fatigue and irritability may be the result of a return to the old lifestyle, with its worries, real or imagined, heavy work schedule, and absence of physical activity and recreation—in short, a repetition of the very set of circumstances that probably triggered the initial acute attack.

Is it not better to be sure than sorry? Within reason, yes. However, a patient cannot keep running in and out of the doctor's office or the hospital emergency department. He or she must learn to exercise judgment and maturity in assessing the significance of various symptoms. Getting into the habit of requiring an electrocardiogram for every ache or pain is the path to cardiac neurosis—in my experience, one of the most difficult of all conditions to cure. If this preoccupation with symptoms that consistently prove to be groundless persists beyond a six-month period or so, and shows no signs of responding to simple reassurance on your part, then it should be mentioned to the family physician or the cardiologist. Psychological treatment may be indicated to relieve the condition before the pattern becomes set.

What About Sexual Activity?
Many postcoronary patients, both male and female, quickly regain their interest in sex after the acute stage of the attack is over and they have returned home to their routine daily activities. The chances are that their level of interest will be the same as previously. This subject is dealt with on pages 312–314, but spouses may have concerns of their own. Most concerns are largely groundless. Unless the heart has been extensively damaged, there is no more danger after the heart attack than there was before it. So don't enter the situation in obvious fear and trepidation. Nothing is more destined to put your partner off and increase feelings of depression, insecurity, and worthlessness.

There are certain medications that, in some patients, may reduce sexual urge. The individual variations are wide, and it is frequently very difficult to distinguish between a true chemical side effect and a host of other less tangible causes. However, there have been reports of reduction in libido following the taking of various drugs used to lower blood pressure, certain beta-blockers, tranquilizers, and antidepressants. If one of these medications is suspected in reducing sexual desire, the matter should be discussed with the prescribing physician. On no account allow your spouse to stop a medication on the grounds of suspicion. It is often relatively easy for the physician to substitute another substance that is equally effective but does not carry the same side effects. While we are on the subject, incidentally, let me remind you that the most common drug that has been shown to reduce sexual appetite is nonprescription—alcohol!

How Can I Prevent Another Attack?

Recognition of dangerous symptoms is one thing; preventing them from appearing is a far more worthwhile goal. What positive steps should you take to help your partner keep from having a further attack? It can be expressed in a phrase: "Give all assistance in efforts to change lifestyle." The previous way of life contained the seeds of the attack. You now have a chance to help alter the situation. This means a prudent diet low in cholesterol and animal fats, a physical-fitness program, a total veto on cigarette smoking (this applies to you, also), and moderation in both work and play.

You will need to accommodate this changed partner. The more accommodation needed, the more you can console yourself with the thought that the rehabilitation is proceeding successfully. You may have to arrange mealtimes to fit in with the exercise sessions. If you can't walk together, then take the trouble to acquaint yourself with the time the workout should take, and then plan accordingly.

Another side effect of increasing fitness is the desire to take up new and sometimes more strenuous leisure activities, such as camping, sailboating, backpacking, and cross-country skiing. Often allied with this is an increased interest in the simpler pleasures; walking in the rain, reading a good novel, taking a fall outing on foot to catch the colors.

It's not always easy to change, even for a good reason. I still recall with crystal clarity the bemused tone with which one of my earliest "successes" described his wife's reaction to his newly awakened yearnings. "You know what she said, Doc?" he intoned sadly. "She said, 'I wish you hadn't changed. We were so happy when you were the way you used to be.'" The way he "used to be" had set the stage for his heart attack!

APPENDIX A: NOMOGRAMS

NOMOGRAM A
To Be Used for Calculating Your Progressing Heart Rate

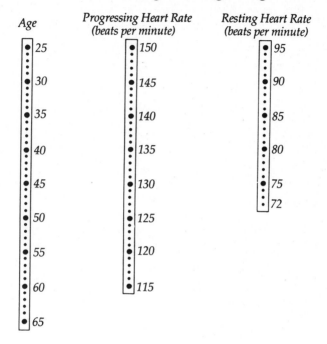

Age

Progressing Heart Rate
(beats per minute)

Resting Heart Rate
(beats per minute)

For those who have completed a stress test without adverse symptoms or who are free from heart disease.

A line joining your resting heart rate and your age will intersect the center column at your progressing heart rate. Resting heart rates below 72 beats per minute should be charted at 72.

To obtain your heart rate (pulse rate) and resting heart rate, see instructions on pages 206–207 and 265–266.

NOMOGRAM B

To Be Used for Calculating Your Training Heart Rate and Your Progressing Heart Rate

Maximum Heart Rate (Symptom Limited)
(beats per minute)

TRAINING HEART RATE
(beats per minute)

PROGRESSING HEART RATE
(beats per minute)

RESTING HEART RATE
(beats per minute)

For those who have not been able to complete a stress test because of the development of adverse symptoms or who have anginal pain, palpitations or breathlessness, etc.

A line joining your resting heart rate and the heart rate at which your symptoms appear, your maximum heart rate (symptom limited), will intersect the center columns at your training heart rate and progressing heart rate. Resting heart rates above 72 beats per minute should be charted at 72.

If the difference between your resting heart rate and your maximum heart rate (symptom limited) is less than 40 beats per minute, you should not attempt the training program in this book, except under medical supervision.

To obtain your heart rate (pulse rate) and resting heart rate, see instructions on pages 206–207 and 265–266.

Appendix A (cont'd)

NOMOGRAM C

Nomogram for Prediction of Maximum Oxygen Intake in Men Aged 25 and 35 Years

Heart Rate
(beats per minute)

Actual
Oxygen Consumption
(millilitres per minute)

Heart Rate	Actual Oxygen Consumption
170	0,800
166	0,900
162	1,000
158	1,100
154	1,200
150	1,300
146	1,400
142	1,500
138	1,600
134	1,700
130	1,800
126	1,900
122	2,000
	2,100
	2,200
	2,300
	2,400
	2,500
	2,600

Age 35   *Age 25*

1,500   1,500

2,000   2,000

2,500   2,500

3,000   3,000

3,500   3,500

4,000   4,000

4,500   4,500

5,000

Maximum
Oxygen Consumption
(millilitres per minute)

A line joining your heart rate and actual oxygen intake will intersect the center line at your maximum oxygen intake.

Appendix A (cont'd)

NOMOGRAM D
Nomogram for Prediction of Maximum Oxygen Intake in Women Aged 25 and 35 Years

Heart Rate
(beats per minute)

- 170
- 166
- 162
- 158
- 154
- 150
- 146
- 142
- 138
- 134
- 130
- 126
- 122

Age
35

Age
25

1,000 1,000

1,500 1,500

2,000 2,000

2,500 2,500

3,000 3,000

3,500 3,500

4,000 4,000

4,500 4,500

5,000

Maximum
Oxygen Consumption
(millilitres per minute)

Actual Oxygen
Consumption
(millilitres
per minute)

- 0,600
- 0,700
- 0,800
- 0,900
- 1,000
- 1,100
- 1,200
- 1,300
- 1,400
- 1,500
- 1,600
- 1,700
- 1,800
- 1,900
- 2,000
- 2,100
- 2,200
- 2,300
- 2,400
- 2,500

A line joining your heart rate and actual oxygen intake will intersect the center line at your maximum oxygen intake.

Appendix A (cont'd)

NOMOGRAM E
Nomogram for Prediction of Maximum Oxygen Intake in Men Aged 45 and 55 Years

Heart Rate
(beats per minute)

Actual
Oxygen Consumption
(millilitres per minute)

- 170
- 166
- 162
- 158
- 154
- 150
- 146
- 142
- 138
- 134
- 130
- 126
- 122

Age 55 Age 45

750 750
1,000 1,000
1,500 1,500
2,000 2,000
2,500 2,500
3,000 3,000
3,500 3,500

Maximum
Oxygen Consumption
(millilitres per minute)

- 0,400
- 0,500
- 0,600
- 0,700
- 0,800
- 0,900
- 1,000
- 1,100
- 1,200
- 1,300
- 1,400
- 1,500
- 1,600
- 1,700
- 1,800
- 1,900
- 2,000
- 2,100
- 2,200
- 2,300

A line joining your heart rate and actual oxygen intake will intersect the center line at your maximum oxygen intake.

Appendix A (cont'd)

NOMOGRAM F

Nomogram for Prediction of Maximum Oxygen Intake in Women Aged 45 and 55 Years

Heart Rate
(beats per minute)

Actual Oxygen
Consumption
(millilitres
per minute)

Maximum
Oxygen Consumption
(millilitres per minute)

A line joining your heart rate and actual oxygen intake will intersect the center line at your maximum oxygen intake.

APPENDIX B: TRAINING TABLES

To be used for determining your exercise prescription, *but* only after careful reading of the text.

If your predicted maximum oxygen consumption (VO_2max) is below 16 milliliters per kilogram per minute, or if you do not actually know what it is, begin at Phase Ia, Level 1. If your maximum oxygen consumption is more than 16 milliliters per kilogram per minute, begin at the appropriate level in Phase Ib (see pages 259–260).

Ideally, in all phases you should plan to exercise 5 times weekly.

Phase Ia
Levels to be taken in sequence.
Level 1   For 2 weeks walk 1 mile (1.6 km) in 30 minutes
Level 2   For 2 weeks walk 1½ miles (2.4 km) in 42 minutes
Level 3   For 2 weeks walk 2 miles (3.2 km) in 50 minutes
Level 4   For 2 weeks walk 2½ miles (4.0 km) in 57½ minutes
When you have completed Phase Ia, progress to Phase Ib, Level 1.

Phase Ib
For instructions on progressing through the levels of Phase Ib, see page 266.

If you begin your exercise program at one of the levels in Phase Ib (see page 259), do not attempt at first the full prescription for your starting level. Instead, start with one-third the starting prescription (e.g., at Level 1, walk 1 mile [1.6 km] in 20 minutes if you are under age 45). After two weeks, progress to two-thirds the starting prescription (e.g., 2 miles [3.2 km] in 40 minutes, if under age 45 and at Level 1) for a further two weeks. Then, provided there are

Appendix B (cont'd)

no adverse symptoms, proceed to the full three miles (4.8 km) in the time prescribed for your starting level. *If you are aged 60 or over, you need go no further than three miles in 45 minutes (Phase Ib, Level 7, column 45 and over), unless you are a lifelong exerciser.*

Phase Ib

Level	Predicted maximum oxygen consumption (milliliters per kilogram per minute)	Distance (miles)	Time (minutes) Under age 45	Time (minutes) 45 and over
1	16.1 to 17.5 mL/kg/min	3	60	63
2	17.6 to 18.4 mL/kg/min	3	57	60
3	18.5 to 21.3 mL/kg/min	3	54	57
4	21.4 to 22.7 mL/kg/min	3	51	54
5	22.8 to 25.6 mL/kg/min	3	48	51
6	25.7 to 28.5 mL/kg/min	3	45	48
7	28.6 + mL/kg/min	3	42	45

The transition stage from walking to jogging can be complicated, and so patients attending the Centre are given the following instructions:

Please note that in the following exercise prescriptions, walking is done at a 15-minutes-per-mile/9:15-minutes-per-kilometer pace, and jogging at 12-minutes-per-mile/7:3-minutes-per-kilometer pace. All speeds for the mile/1.6-kilometer and 3-mile/4.8-kilometer distances are rounded off to the nearest minute or quarter-minute. It is essential to keep as closely as possible to the 15-minutes-per-mile/9:15-minutes-per-kilometer pace for walking, and the 12-

Appendix B (cont'd)

minutes-per-mile/7:3-minutes-per-kilometer pace for jogging. The 13½-minutes-per-mile/8:3-minutes-per-kilometer pace is repeated in the tables so as to effect a smoother transition from half-lap (100-meter/110-yard) jogs to whole-lap (200-meter/220-yard) jogs.

1) 14½-minute-mile/9-minute-kilometer (43½ minutes for 3 miles/4.8 kilometers). Alternate 3½ laps walking with a half-lap jogging for a total of 24 laps to give 3 miles/4.8 kilometers.

2) 14-minute-mile/8:45-minute-kilometer (42 minutes for 3 miles/4.8 kilometers). Alternate 1½ laps walking with a half-lap jogging for a total of 24 laps to give 3 miles/4.8 kilometers.

3a) 13½-minute-mile/8:30-minute-kilometer (40½ minutes for 3 miles/4.8 kilometers). Alternate half-lap walk with half-lap jog for a total of 24 laps to give 3 miles/4.8 kilometers.

3b) 13½-minute-mile/8:30-minute-kilometer (40½ minutes for 3 miles/4.8 kilometers). Alternate one lap walk with one lap jog for a total of 24 laps to give 3 miles/4.8 kilometers.

4) 13-minute-mile/8-minute-kilometer (39 minutes for 3 miles/4.8 kilometers). Alternate half-lap walk with 1½ laps jogging for a total of 24 laps to give 3 miles/4.8 kilometers.

5) 12-minute-mile/7.3-minute-kilometer (36 minutes for 3 miles/4.8 kilometers). Jog the entire distance.

If you don't attend the Centre's program, but have access to a 200- or 400-meter/220- or 440-yard track, then you should adhere to the above instructions.

However, if you are using the sidewalk or park as your training course, you will have to use a slightly different approach. Your first most important task is to familiarize

Appendix B (cont'd)

yourself with the 15 minutes-per-mile (9.15-minutes-per-kilometer) walking pace and then with the 12-minutes-per-mile (7:30-minutes-per-kilometer) jogging pace. The latter is equivalent to jogging 110 yards/100 meters in 45 seconds. Once you have mastered this, then the five stages outlined above can be expressed as follows:

1) 14½-minute-mile/9-minute-kilometer (43½ minutes for 3 miles/4.8 kilometers). Alternate 6½ minutes walk (700 meters/770 yards at a 15-minute-mile/9:15-minute-kilometer pace) with a 45-second jog (at a 12-minute-mile/7:30-minute-kilometer pace) for a total of 3 miles/4.8 kilometers.

2) 14-minute-mile/8:45-minute-kilometer (42 minutes for 3 miles/4.8 kilometers). Alternate 2:45 walk (330 yards/300 meters), with 45-second jog (110 yards/100 meters) for a total of 3 miles/4.8 kilometers.

3a) 13½-minute-mile/8:30-minute-kilometer (40½ minutes for 3 miles/4.8 kilometers). Alternate a 56-second walk (110 yards/100 meters) with a 45-second jog (110 yards/100 meters) for a total of 3 miles/4.8 kilometers.

3b) 13½-minute-mile/8:30-minute-kilometer (40½ minutes for 3 miles/4.8 kilometers). Alternate 1:53 walk (220 yards/200 meters), with a 90-second jog (220 yards/200 meters) for a total of 3 miles/4.8 kilometers.

Appendix B (cont'd)

Phase II

For instructions on progressing through the levels of Phase II, see pages 260–261.

Level	Age Under 45				Age 45–59		
	Distance (miles)	Distance (meters)*	Time (minutes)	Approx. Pace (mins./ mile)	Distance (miles)	Time (minutes)	Approx. Pace (mins./ mile)
1	3	4828	43½	14½	3	43½	14½
2	3	4828	42	14	3	42	14
3	3	4828	40½	13½(a)	3	40½	13½(a)
4	3	4828	40½	13½(b)	3	40½	13½(b)
5	3	4828	39	13	3	39	13
6	3	4828	36	12	3	36	12
7	3½	5230	39	12	3½	39	12
8	3½	5633	42	12	3½	42	12
9	3½	6035	45	12	3½	45	12
10	4	6437	48	12	4	48	12
11	4	6437	46	11½			
12	4	6437	44	11			
13	4	6437	42	10½	*Metric equivalents		
14	4	6437	40	10	are approximate.		

After Phase II, Level 11, you may progress to Phase III.

Phase III

For more instructions on progressing through the levels of Phase III, see page 261.

Level	Distance (miles)	Distance (meters)	Age Under 45 Time (minutes)	Age 45–59 Time (minutes)
1	4¼	6800	42½	51
2	4½	7200	45	54
3	4¾	7600	47½	57
4	5	8000	50	60

APPENDIX C: HEAT SAFETY INDEX

Heat Safety Index

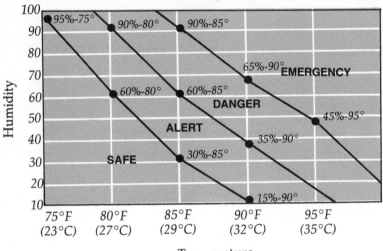

APPENDIX D: WIND CHILL FACTORS

Wind Speed mph (km/h)*	Temperature °F (°C)*				
Calm	40(5)	35(2)	30(−1)	25(−4)	20(−7)
5(8)	35	30	25	20	15
10(16)	30	20	15	10	5
15(24)	25	15	10	0	−5
20(32)	20	10	5	0	−10
25(40)	15	10	0	−5	−15

Do not exercise out of doors when the wind chill factor is below the level indicated to the left of the heavy line.

*Metric equivalents are approximate.

Source: Adapted from a chart by Dr. Charles Egan.

APPENDIX E: FITNESS FOR SPORTS

You need to be fit to take part in games and sports. A good guide to your cardiovascular ability to participate is the level of your performance on the training tables.*

To participate in: Sport		You need to be able to walk/jog 3 miles (4.8 km) in:
		(min.)
Archery		60–57
Badminton	— social	39
	— more vigorously	30–24
Basketball	— recreational	39
	— game	30–24
Bowling		54
Canoeing	— leisurely	60–54
	— vigorously	45–36
Cycling	— 8 mph	60
	— 10 mph	45
	— 12 mph	36
	— 15 mph	30
Gardening	— raking	72
	— mowing	42
	— digging	36
Golf	— using power cart	60
	— pulling a club cart	48
	— carrying clubs	42
Handball	— easy	36
	— more vigorously	30
Hockey, Field		30
Horseback riding	— walking	60
	— trotting	42
	— galloping	33
Ice skating	— leisurely	45
	— quickly	36–30

Appendix E (cont'd)

To participate in:		You need to be able to walk/jog 3 miles (4.8 km) in:
Sport		
		(min.)
Skiing	— cross country (very leisurely)	42–36
	— cross country (4 mph)	33
	— cross country (5 mph)	30
	— cross country (8 mph)	21
	— downhill (easily)	42–36
	— downhill (vigorously)	36–30
Snowshoeing		30–24
Soccer (depending on position and level of play)		54–36
Squash		25–18
Swimming (assuming a reasonably proficient swimmer, and optimal water temperature of 82-86°F [28-30°C)		
	Breast stroke	30–27
	Crawl stroke	33–30
	Back stroke	33–30
	Side stroke	36–33
	Treading water	60–54
Tennis	— doubles	48
	— singles	33

*Values are based on a 150-lb (70-kg) person.

APPENDIX F: PAR-Q AND YOU

The Physical Activity Readiness Questionnaire (PAR-Q) is designed to help you help yourself. Many health benefits are associated with regular exercise, and the completion of PAR-Q is a sensible first step to take if you are planning to increase the amount of physical activity in your life.

For most people physical activity should not pose any problem or hazard. PAR-Q has been designed to identify the small number of adults for whom physical activity might be inappropriate or those who should have medical advice concerning the type of activity most suitable for them.

Common sense is your best guide in answering these few questions. Please read them carefully and check (✓) the ❑ YES or ❑ NO opposite the question if it applies to you.

Yes No

❑   ❑ 1. Has a doctor ever said that you have a heart condition and recommended only medically supervised activity?

❑   ❑ 2. Do you have chest pain brought on by physical activity?

❑   ❑ 3. Have you developed chest pain in the past month?

❑   ❑ 4. Do you tend to lose consciousness or fall over as a result of dizziness?

❑   ❑ 5. Do you have a bone or joint problem that could be aggravated by the proposed physical activity?

❑   ❑ 6. Has a doctor ever recommended medication for your blood pressure or a heart condition?

❑   ❑ 7. Are you aware through your own experience, or a doctor's advice, of any other physical reason against your exercising without medical supervision?

Note: If you have a temporary illness, such as a common cold, or are not feeling well at this time—**postpone**.

Appendix F (cont'd)

If you answered YES to one or more questions

If you have not recently done so, consult your personal physician by telephone or in person BEFORE increasing your physical activity and/or taking a fitness appraisal. Tell your physician what questions you answered YES to on PAR-Q or present your PAR-Q copy.

Programs

After medical evaluation, seek advice from your physician as to your suitability for:

- unrestricted physical activity starting off easily and progressing gradually
- restricted or supervised activity to meet your specific needs, at least on an initial basis. Check in your community for special programs or services.

If you answered NO to all questions

If you answered PAR-Q accurately, you have reasonable assurance of your present suitability for:

- A GRADUATED EXERCISE PROGRAM—a gradual increase in proper exercise promotes good fitness development while minimizing or eliminating discomfort.
- A FITNESS APPRAISAL—the Canadian Standardized Test of Fitness (CSTF).

Postpone

If you have a temporary minor illness, such as a common cold.

Source: Revised Physical Activity Readiness Questionnaire (PAR-Q). PAR-Q Validation Report. British Columbia Ministry of Health/Produced by the British Columbia Ministry of Health and the Department of National Health & Welfare. From Canadian Standardized Test of Fitness (CSTF) Operations Manual, 3rd Ed. With the permission of Fitness Canada, Fitness and Amateur Sport Canada, Ottawa, 1986.

APPENDIX G: HOW TO ESTIMATE YOUR RATE OF STEPPING

How to Estimate Your Rate of Stepping, the Resulting Energy Cost, and Target Heart Rate from Your Weight and Age

Rate of Stepping (steps per min.)	Energy Cost of Stepping (milliliters of oxygen)

MALE

Weight lbs. (kg.) AGE	110 (49.9)	120 (54.4)	130 (59.0)	140 (63.5)	150 (68.0)	160 (72.6)	170 (77.1)	180 (81.6)	190 (86.2)	200 (90.7)	210 (95.3)	220 (99.8)
20-29	120	120	120	126	126	126	126	126	126	126	126	126
	1570	1690	1813	2018	2143	2273	2398	2524	2653	2779	2908	3034
30-39	108	114	114	114	114	114	114	114	114	120	120	120
	1437	1618	1734	1848	1962	2079	2192	2307	2423	2658	2781	2901
40-49	96	96	96	102	102	102	102	102	102	102	102	102
	1304	1400	1498	1679	1781	1885	1987	2089	2193	2295	2400	2502
50-60	78	78	78	78	78	78	84	84	84	84	84	84
	1105	1183	1262	1340	1418	1498	1679	1763	1849	1933	2018	2103

FEMALE

Weight lbs. (kg.) AGE	80 (36.3)	90 (40.8)	100 (45.4)	110 (49.9)	120 (54.4)	130 (59.0)	140 (63.5)	150 (68.0)	160 (72.6)	170 (77.1)	180 (81.6)	190 (86.2)
20-29	96	102	102	102	102	108	108	108	108	108	108	108
	974	1125	1229	1331	1433	1616	1724	1832	1942	2050	2158	2268
30-39	96	96	102	102	102	102	102	108	108	108	108	108
	974	1070	1229	1331	1433	1537	1639	1832	1942	2050	2158	2268
40-49	84	84	84	90	90	90	90	90	90	90	96	96
	877	961	1047	1198	1288	1380	1469	1560	1652	1742	1288	2038
50-60	60	60	60	60	60	60	60	60	60	60	60	60
	684	744	805	865	925	986	1046	1106	1168	1228	1288	1349

Appendix F (cont'd)

Target Heart Rates
(age-related) after 3–5 minutes of stepping

Age (Years)	Heart Rate (Beats/min.)
20–29	160/min.
30–39	150/min.
40–49	140/min.
50–59	130/min.
60–70	120/min.

APPENDIX H:

Cholesterol Screening and Treatment Guidelines
Age: 30 years and over
(Adapted from NCEP Report, 1994)

Level	Blood Cholesterol	Risk	Action
1	Total-C ≤ 5.2 mmol/L (200 mg/dL)	Desirable	Recheck within 5 years or with physical examination.
2	Total-C 5.2–6.2 mmol/L (200–239 mg/dL)	Borderline High	Restrict saturated fats; advise physical activity program; recheck Total-C and HDL-C in 1 year.
	2a: HDL-C of 0.9 mmol/L (35 mg/dL) or less and fewer than two other risk factors,[1] goal is to keep Total-C below 6.2 mmol/L (240 mg/dL); LDL-C below 4.1 mmol/L (160 mg/dL); and HDL-C at or above 0.9 mmol/L (35 mg/dL).		
	2b: *Without* CHD and with two or more risk factors, goal is to keep Total-C at or below 5.2 mmol/L (200 mg/dL); LDL-C below 3.4 mmol/L (130 mg/dL); and HDL-C at or above 0.9 mmol/L (35 mg/dL). *With* CHD, LDL-C goal is 2.6 mmol/L (100 mg/dL).	High Risk	Check fasting triglycerides, LDL[2] and HDL[3]-C. If abnormal, Step I of AHA diet.[4] Advise physical activity program. Once goal is attained, maintain diet and exercise, and check blood cholesterol at appropriate intervals. If goal is not attained, Step II of AHA diet.[4] Physical activity program. If goal still not attained, physician may consider drug therapy.
3	Greater than 6.2 mmol/L (240 mg/dL); *with or without* CHD risk factors, goal is to keep Total-C below 5.2 mmol/L (200 mg/dL); LDL-C below 2.6 mmol/L (100 mg/dL); and HDL-C above 0.9 mmol/L (35 mg/dL).	High Risk	As for 2b, although some physicians may wish to go straight to Step II diet, or in presence of CHD, to drug therapy.

[1]**Risk Factors**
- male gender
- age (men ≥ 45 years; women ≥ 55 years or premature menopause without hormone replacement therapy)
- family history of premature CHD (definite heart attack or sudden death before 55 years of age in father or brother, or before 65 years of age in mother or sister)
- hypertension (≥ 140/90 mm Hg)
- current cigarette smoking
- diabetes
- history of stroke
- severe obesity (30% overweight)
- HDL-C ≤ 0.9 mmol/L (35 mg/dL). If the HDL-C is ≤1.6 mmol/L (60 mg/dL), subtract one risk factor (because high HDL-C levels decrease CHD risk).

---

[2]**LDL-C:** This is not measured directly but is calculated from your Total-C, Triglycerides, and HDL-C as follows:

$$\text{LDL-C (mmol/L)} = \text{Total C} - \text{HDL-C} - \frac{\text{Triglycerides (mg/dL)}}{2.2}$$

$$\text{LDL-C (mg/dL)} = \text{Total C} - \text{HDL-C} - \frac{\text{Triglycerides (mg/dL)}}{5}$$

	Desirable LDL-C Levels
No risk factors	≤ 4.2 mmol/L (160 mg/dL)
Two or more risk factors	≤ 3.4 mmol/L (130 mg/dL)
With CHD	≤ 2.6 mmol/L (100 mg/dL)

---

[3]**HDL-C:**

	Desirable HDL-C Levels
All Subjects	≥ 0.9 mmol/L (35 mg/dL)

*Total-C to HDL-C Ratio $\frac{\text{Total-C}}{\text{HDL-C}}$

*This ratio is not included in the NCEP recommendations, but data from the Framingham study strongly support its use as a CHD predictor.

Women	Men	Risk
2.5	3.4	½ average
4.4	5.1	average
6.4	6.8	2X average
7.5	7.8	3X average

---

[4]**The American Heart Association Recommended Low-Fat Diet:**

Nutrient	Recommended Intake	
	Step I Diet	**Step II Diet**
Total Fat	Less than 30% of Total Calories	
Saturated Fatty Acids	Less than 10% of Total Calories	Less than 7% of Total Calories
Polyunsaturated Fatty Acids	Up to 10% of Total Calories	
Monounsaturated Fatty Acids	10 to 15% of Total Calories	
Carbohydrates	50 to 60% of Total Calories	
Protein	10 to 20% of Total Calories	
Cholesterol	Less than 300 mg/day	Less than 200 mg/day
Total Calories	To achieve and maintain desirable weight	

Index